Let Faith Grow

RUNNING THROUGH ADVERSITY

BEN HINTON

STREAMLINE BOOKS

LET FAITH GROW

Running Through Adversity

Copyright © 2023 by Ben Hinton

All rights reserved.

Scriptures taken from the Holy Bible, New International Version®, NIV®. Copyright © 1973, 1978, 1984, 2011 by Biblica, Inc.™ Used by permission of Zondervan. All rights reserved worldwide. www.zondervan.com The "NIV" and "New International Version" are trademarks registered in the United States Patent and Trademark Office by Biblica, Inc.™

Scripture quotations marked (NLT) are taken from the *Holy Bible*, New Living Translation, copyright ©1996, 2004, 2015 by Tyndale House Foundation. Used by permission of Tyndale House Publishers, Carol Stream, Illinois 60188. All rights reserved.

Cover design by Will Severns

Streamline Books | www.StreamlineBooksPublishing.com

Paperback ISBN: 9-798-8508-9389-7

Hardcover ISBN: 9-798-8508-9412-2

July 11th, 2023

Dedication

I want to thank first and foremost my Lord and Savior, Jesus Christ. I want to dedicate this book and any of this book's success to you, Lord. Last year, I came to the realization that my biggest fear in life was when success came my way, I'd be stealing His success. In other words, I want to always remember to remain humble.

I also want to dedicate this book to my wife, Crystal Amy Hinton. Thank you for giving me the greatest gift of fatherhood. Something we both always wanted was a family. It has been something we have had to fight for in so many ways and in ways that neither of us would have ever imagined. I can speak for both of us in saying that it was worth it all with the blessing of our two girls, Brielle and Charlie. I have been so thankful to watch them develop as individuals and as sisters. I always wanted siblings growing up, and I have been able to see that loving relationship blossom between the two of them despite their five-year age difference. They are my "why." At times, I can be obsessed, a pain in the butt, and over-analytical of my goals. At the end of the day, I want to look back and say I lived my life to show them how to chase their dreams, show up, and grow despite any and ALL external factors in life. My girls' growth has been amazing to watch at their young age.

To Brielle and Charlie, your mother and I can't wait for your growth to only continue.

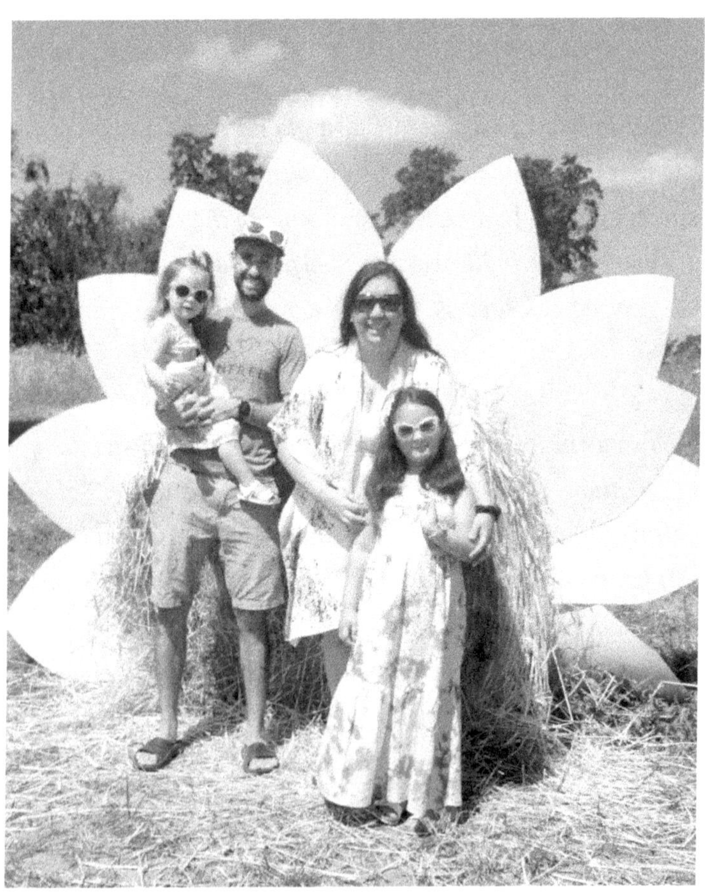

Contents

PART THREE
EMPTYING THE TANK IN LOVE

DR. MATTHEW POREMBA

Foreword

In the labyrinth of life, we often find ourselves confronted with unforeseen obstacles that test the limits of our physical and mental endurance. These challenges come in various forms—some arise from external circumstances beyond our control, while others emerge from the depths of our own minds, seemingly insurmountable. Yet, it is precisely in these moments of profound struggle that the human spirit reveals its most extraordinary strength.

The book you hold in your hands is a testament to the indomitable nature of the human will—a story that will illuminate the transformative power of perseverance, resilience, and unwavering determination. Within these pages, you will embark on a remarkable journey alongside an individual who has confronted adversity head-on, refusing to be defined by his limitations.

Physical challenges can manifest in countless ways,

whether it be battling a debilitating illness, recovering from a traumatic injury, or striving to overcome the seemingly insurmountable odds of an athletic pursuit. The story contained herein will introduce you to a remarkable individual who has faced these trials with unparalleled courage and conviction. Through his account, you will witness the boundless potential of the human body to heal, adapt, and emerge stronger than ever before.

But the challenges we face extend beyond the realm of the physical. The human mind, with its intricate labyrinth of thoughts and emotions, can become a battleground of its own. Within these pages, you will find an individual who has bravely embarked on the journey of self-discovery and emotional healing. His tale will inspire you to confront your own doubts and fears, reminding you that triumph over mental challenges is possible, even when the road ahead seems insurmountable.

As you delve into this narrative, you will bear witness to the struggles and setbacks that this individual encountered. The path to triumph is not linear —it twists and turns, testing the limits of our resolve. But in this story, you will find the glimmers of hope, the defining moments of breakthrough, and the relentless pursuit of a brighter future. This tale will serve as a guiding light, illuminating the way forward when the darkness threatens to overwhelm us.

Through the power of storytelling, we have the privilege of experiencing the profound impact that determination, resilience, and an unwavering belief in oneself can have on our lives. The father, husband and man showcased within this book is not extraordinary with supernatural abilities; he is an ordinary person who has tapped into an extraordinary reserve of strength within themselves.

In sharing his story, he invites us to embark on our own personal odysseys, empowering us to face our challenges head-on. His triumphs remind us that, regardless of the obstacles we face, we possess the capacity to rise above, to evolve, and to transcend our limitations. The true essence of victory lies not solely in achieving the desired outcome, but rather in the unwavering pursuit of our dreams, in the relentless fight against adversity, and in the knowledge that our inner fortitude can carry us to unimaginable heights.

So, dear reader, as you turn these pages, immerse yourself in the triumphs and tribulations that lie within. Let this story of courage, resilience, and ultimate success ignite the flame within your own heart. May you find solace in his experience, strength in his perseverance, and inspiration in his unyielding belief in the human spirit.

For in the face of adversity, it is not merely about surviving—it is about flourishing. It is about embracing the triumph within.

Preface

Thank you so much for picking up *Let Faith Grow*. I'd like to take a minute, just sit right there . . . (Does anyone else get that *Fresh Prince of Bel Air* vibe going with that?) In my opinion, mental health has become the forefront of conversation in our society ever since 2020. I am sure you would probably agree. One of the things about mental health is the pressure it creates. The labels, the stress, and everything else all snowballs and keeps getting bigger. I believe that lives will be transformed when we SHARE our faith and do not push our faith. The longest relationship we will ever be involved with for the duration of our lives is the relationship we have with ourselves. So, I have truly learned to believe that when we let our faith grow it can help crush the pressure to perform.

Do you agree the pressure to perform is a huge part of our society's mental health struggles? We are wearing more "hats" now than we ever did. I don't know a man, woman, or child that can't relate to this. Am I an expert in mental health? I am not! I eventually graduated with a bachelor's in history from the University of Pittsburgh. In particular, I studied with an emphasis on the effects of the Triangular trade in the United States. Is this book going to be a history lesson? No, definitely not. My minor was geology and I struggled with that, so there will be no talk about rocks (goals in stone on the other hand).

What I am going to share with you is my faith through my life experiences, particularly my lived experience from 2013 to the present time of this book. I have developed principles based on my own experience (experience being our greatest teacher). Sometimes the lessons learned come from the insight of my mentors as well as through trial and error. This is not a workbook for your life, but I do hope it is a useful tool. I hope that some principals—if not all the ones I share in this book—can help you grow; in doing so, it will help you crush the pressure to perform. This is not a workbook because I think the principles can help you organically shift things in your life for the better. In a way, the "work" has already been set before you. From my faith perspective, I do believe we have already won. We are already accepted. I want you to read this book so you can establish your principles, and bring more awareness to your personal life—emotionally, socially, and physically. The journey is tough regardless, but we can grow through what we go through.

When I am hopefully 90+ years old, I do not want to live a life of regret. I believe that a life of regret means you simply have years and years built on top of never taking any action. If you get anything from the overall scope of this book, I want you to remember that "Failure is an option, regret is not." I don't want to live a life of regret, and I don't want you to live a life of regret either.

Before you dive into this book, I want to make you aware of a few more things. The first is the subtitle: "Running through Adversity." I don't want this book to come off as a guide for runners or just a book for "athletes." My story, my experiences, and my goals do stem from running and athletics. Yet, I want you to be able to carry my principles into your life, your career, and your goals however that manifests. Whatever that burning desire or goal is for you, I want you to implement these principles into your life. I hope it affirms and builds principles you already have.

The reason why this book is not a workbook and doesn't come off as self-help (live your best, be your best) is because I want this book to inspire you to and excite you to the point that you borrow these principles and make them your own. In other words, don't reinvent the wheel, but let some or all of the principles become a part of you and grow! I hope that down the line I hear new principles from a speaker, or an author, and maybe they mention I was a part of their growth through this book. Another way to say it is, "Excitement can be caught, not taught." Yes, I hope that this book motivates you. More than that, I want to inspire you. I have learned that motivation is great, but it is just like the remote car starter. You're looking out the window and you get the car heated up and ready (motivation), but it doesn't go anywhere until you get out the door, put your foot to the gas, and drive. That is the inspiration. That is the action part. I know I have been like that many times in my life where I became personally motivated, but didn't go anywhere! That will actually drive you crazy. It's like how they say the definition of crazy is beating your head against the wall again and again, and expecting different results. Have you maybe experienced that? Being motivated, but not getting any closer to the areas you want to improve in your life? Well, I hope this book inspires you.

Lastly, before you dive into the book, remember that I believe in YOU! My personal philosophy can be summed up as: "Be encouraged everyday, to encourage others is to encourage ourselves, to love others is to love ourselves." I love you whether I know you or not. Also please highlight this: "Have your best today." Life is a series of ebbs and flows. Jim Rohn said it best: "After expansion is recession, after recession is expansion. To think differently is naive." So let's stop being naive—let's stop trying to have the BEST DAY EVER, every single day. Let's be consistently consistent and have our best today. Let today be its best day. That should take pressure off the "I'll be happy when" mentality. Choose happiness for today.

Now that you know a little bit more about the title of this book, I am going to be vulnerable and share my story now . . . Side note: "True strength is being vulnerable." Stay in touch, share, and please have a conversation with those around you if this book impacts you in a positive way. Without further ado, I present to you *Let Faith Grow: Running Through Adversity*. Enjoy!

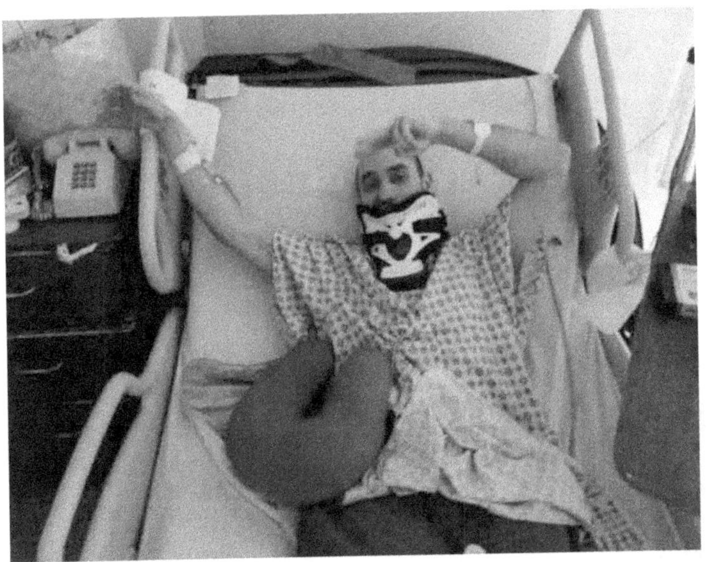

In the hospital after sustaining a traumatic brain injury in 2013.

Let Faith Grow

Introduction

I am so glad you picked up *Let Faith Grow: Running Through Adversity*. My name is Ben Hinton. Not only am I a marathon runner, but I'm also a Christian, a husband to a wonderful wife, a dad to two beautiful little girls, and from my youth into my twenties, I was an aspiring NBA player. (Any Pittsburgh sports fans out there?) We are huge Penguins and Steelers fans. But all of these facts are only a glimpse into my story.

I didn't start running until 2013, which was exactly eight weeks after I sustained a serious brain injury.

Yup, you read that right. Merely eight weeks after a severe, debilitating brain injury, I ran my first half marathon.

I am not sharing this to garner your sympathy or pity. Rather, I'm sharing to provide insight into how adversity has shaped my life.

Let me give you a quick recap:

- I was born June 11, 1986 to a single, workaholic (and alcoholic as I'd come to find out) mother. Six weeks later, I was diagnosed with herpes meningoencephalitis, which meant that the thin layer of tissue covering my brain and my brain itself were both inflamed. At the time, the survival rates for the disease were extremely low. But, thank you, Jesus—I survived.
- As I grew up, I remember my mom calling me her "miracle baby." I didn't have siblings, and although I knew she meant well, that reminder of being the only child (let alone one who survived a disease that's difficult to endure) created a pressure to perform. From a young age, I knew about my diagnosis, and I was thankful to be alive. But my diagnosis also meant that I had the added pressure of comparison. I knew I had differences; I was smaller than other kids my age. In turn, I felt like I always had to prove myself to others. By no means do I blame my mom for any of this—I realized later on that this was a narrative I had told myself for years. I just wanted to be her "perfect child".
- I received a basketball hoop from one of my mom's boyfriends early on (I would say around six years old). It was sturdy and

extended its full six feet in the basement. I was hooked, and so I'd spend hours locked away in the house, just playing hoops. Basketball gave me a sense of purpose, so much so that I decided I was going to play in the NBA. I was going to earn enough money to support my mom. The pressure (I put on myself) to become an NBA player only began to grow and would eventually consume me. I grew up living in the results I wanted (NBA) and didn't enjoy the effort (day-to-day love). I wouldn't understand how much pressure this was internally until I was an adult! This is a theme throughout the book.

- In 3rd grade, mom and I moved to Pittsburgh. That's when her alcoholism became quite noticeable. I missed a lot of elementary school, and there were days where I'd call my mom's employer to call in sick for her.

- Around 7th grade, I was playing pickup games at the YMCA with some kids and teens. We did this all the time. A friend of mine accidentally poked me in the right eye. It was so minor that I didn't give it much thought, but as time wore on, my eye became red and irritated. It was initially misdiagnosed—I was given steroid drops as the doctors thought it was pink eye. It turns out the herpes virus was attacking my retina.

Eventually, I was diagnosed with retinal necrosis. Being poked in the eye could have been just enough to trigger the virus. It was a very rare diagnosis, especially for a child. It took a while for the infectious disease doctors to grasp the cause. No one connected the initial dots that the HSV virus I was born with could spread due to the stress of being poked in the eye. The virus I was born with doesn't have a cure. Up until that point, my lower stress levels played a major role in keeping the virus dormant. Doctors were able to treat the virus, but at a cost—a permanent retina detachment.

- At sixteen years old, I began losing sight in my left eye. We discovered the retinal necrosis was spreading and had started attacking the left eye. I had so many questions and went through months of treatment. Eventually, my vision returned to my left eye.

- On January 9, 2013, while home alone, I sustained a traumatic brain injury by falling down a flight of stairs. I don't remember falling at all. It was a blur. I just remember the date: January 9, 2013. To this day, no one knows how or why I fell. My fiancée (now wife as of July 6, 2013) found me in the basement when she came home from work. She called my childhood best friend,

Matthew Poremba (who was an ER doctor), and brought me to the hospital, where I ended up staying for eighteen days. I was home alone, at the bottom of the basement steps, for roughly 4-5 hours after the fall. God was with me!!!

- From 2014-2015, I received outpatient brain rehabilitation. I was in therapy for thirty-five to forty hours a week, Monday to Friday. Working on myself was my job in my late twenties. I had to start ALL over—forget making a living for my future family. This became a lot of personal pressure. I was so fortunate to be able to be in the outpatient clinic. How I didn't need inpatient rehab is a blessing, due to the injuries I sustained. My cognitive functions were affected greatly. The left side of my body's balance system (vestibular) was shattered. I also lost permanent hearing in my left ear from the impact of the fall. Again, only eight weeks after the brain injury, I ran my first half marathon. Backtracking a little—a desire to be in the Olympics came about in August 2012. I can tell you one thing—running was not exactly the sport I thought I would pursue. After my brain injury, my balance system was shattered. I lost permanent hearing in my left ear, and I already couldn't see out of my right eye since I was 13. Who would have thought that I would ever have the desire to run 26.2 miles at an elite level after January 9, 2013? Isn't God funny?

- In 2015, my vision to run in the Olympics grew. I ran with an ambition to be in the Olympic Trials during 2016 and 2020 without success. But the 2024 Olympic trials are quickly approaching . . . I haven't given up on my vision; I'm still trying, growing, and showing up.

This book focuses on my life experience as an athlete—a runner to be more specific. If you're not an athlete or runner, that's okay, too. Thanks for joining me on this journey. The principles in this book will still be applicable towards you and your passions, pursuits, or endeavors.

Over the next twelve chapters, *Let Faith Grow* will be your guide to warming up, leaning forward, and racing through life to the best of your ability. This book will equip your mind with the tools needed to perform well in your day-to-day, especially throughout every single training run or race that you complete. You'll learn more about my journey and how I have overcome adversity. But most importantly, my hope is that your faith will grow.

PART ONE

Warming Up

"'For I know the plans I have for you,' declares the Lord, 'plans to prosper you and not to harm you, plans to give you hope and a future.'"

— JEREMIAH 29:11

CHAPTER 1

Goals in Stone, Plans in Sand

RACE: 2013 PITTSBURGH HALF MARATHON;
RESULT: 2:10:17, MILE PACE: 9:56/MI

One thing I tell athletes (and myself) is you want to dream. You want to dream so big that God has to get involved. Let me further explain what I mean by this.

Often, we get stuck, or rather fixated, on setting two types of goals. The first type of goal is unrealistic, and let me tell you—the world makes sure to shout at us about how unrealistic it is. The other type of goal is too realistic, maybe too calculated—we will hit it regardless of how much effort we put in.

As Christians, and especially if you are an athlete, the ultimate goal or purpose of anything we do is for God's purpose. We should desire to set goals where God's purpose is so much bigger than ourselves, because ultimately we know God is not constrained by things of the world.

When you have a *goal in stone* that's bigger than

you, it always leads to an opportunity for you to learn how to pivot with purpose and let God lead you. He will take care of the details.

For me, the idea of *goals in stone* started in 2013 with the Pittsburgh Half Marathon. Unlike the other runners, I was only eight weeks into recovery after a serious brain injury.

I wanted to finish the race. My time didn't matter— I didn't feel the need to put extra pressure on myself. If I walked a little, no big deal. Somehow, in some way, I knew that I needed to finish every step of the 13.1 miles of the race.

You see, I had signed up for the Pittsburgh Half Marathon in 2012 right before my brain injury happened on January 9, 2013. After being in the hospital for eighteen days (eleven of which I don't even remember), my doctor told me running the race was unrealistic. I couldn't hear out of my left ear; I couldn't see out of my right eye. My doctor had concerns about my physical well-being, and under- standably so.

One of the first things I do remember after regaining consciousness was walking into a doctor's office, and the doctor saying, "Wow, we didn't think you were going to make it." Hearing that over and over again takes a toll on you mentally and emotionally.

So, originally after hearing the medical staff voice their concerns, I decided to not run the Pittsburgh Half Marathon.

I told myself, "The doctors know what they're talking about. Besides, I just experienced a significant brain injury. I need more time to allow my brain and my body to heal and recover."

That's what was realistic, right? Would my body and brain heal?

I called the Pittsburgh Half Marathon office and explained my situation. I asked the lady who answered the phone how I could transfer my bib and get my money back. To get a refund, she said that I needed to transfer my bib and that someone would have to buy it from me. Otherwise, I'd be out $100 and lose the chance to do something I wanted to do.

At that moment, the light bulb came on. I realized that man (the doctor) had given me a *prognosis*, but only God (the ultimate doctor) knew my true *outcome*. He has already determined it. The half marathon was an opportunity that God created just for me. I had no idea how truly life-changing that realization would be.

A goal had been *set in stone*. From then on, a fire grew within me. I knew I was going to run the half marathon. Nothing anyone else had to say would prevent me from achieving my goals. I had gained confidence in myself.

However, I still had hurdles to overcome. First, I had to adapt to hearing loss in one ear. The hearing in my right ear was so much better that it tried to over-compensate for the hearing loss in my left ear. When I went to public places, my anxiety skyrocketed because of all the audio I picked up around me. Noise would constantly bounce off objects and people. This condition, otherwise referred to as sensory overload, can cause panic attacks and make you feel lost and lonely. Secondly, with my limited eyesight, my doctor didn't want me to run surrounded by a sea of other runners due to safety concerns. I was at risk of falling for six months. The left side of my vestibular system was permanently shattered. He worried I would miss visual cues from others around me and as a result, trip and fall. I decided I'd stay on the right side of the course, out of the way of the main channel of runners. I told my doctor not to worry—I wouldn't run. I'd walk if I had to walk. But deep down, I knew I was going to run.

On race day, I didn't have a time to beat or a personal record to set. I simply ran the race. When I finished the half marathon, it was one of the best feelings in my entire life. I felt so free, knowing this was only a benchmark of things that were not controlled by my brain injury. It was only the starting line of things that I could actually accomplish. With God, anything seemed possible.

After the race, I didn't know what to do. Could I go back to just being the guy that survived a major brain injury?

No, it became impossible to go back to that reality. My adversity and my story became a way to share my faith with others. I knew that I could pursue dreams so big that God's fingerprints—or in other words, His evidence—would be all over them.

For a greater part of my life, I didn't understand what *plans in sand* meant. It's a fine line of being confident while also pivoting with purpose. Sometimes in life, you have to be confident enough to pivot with purpose. Don't pivot just to pivot. Set your goals in stone, but make your plans in sand because they are fickle. Those plans can change more quickly than when a seashell comes in during high tide; you don't have a chance to catch the shell before the ocean takes it out and hides it beneath the surface.

I figured out *plans in sand* in 2014 when I ran my second half marathon and I significantly improved my time. I had a bigger goal; my plans pivoted. We sometimes put our goals on a pedestal and hold them too tightly. We can't relax and we beat ourselves up when we don't reach them. But, we have to learn that it's okay to pivot with purpose and slow down. Pivoting gives you an opportunity to build more confidence and practice your effort. Always put your *goals in stone*. Put your *plans in sand* and wait for the Lord. He alone will guide and direct your path.

"The desert and the parched land shall be glad; the wilderness shall rejoice and blossom. Like the crocus; it will burst into bloom; it will rejoice greatly and shout for joy."

— ISAIAH 35:1-2

CHAPTER 2
Leader of One

After running the Pittsburgh Half Marathon in 2013, I kept training and improving. By the fall of 2014, I saw so much personal improvement at the 2014 Buffalo Creek Half Marathon compared to that previous run in 2013. My form looked good, my pace improved, and my confidence soared higher than ever. This resulted in me setting a *goal in stone* of wanting to run and qualify for the Boston Marathon. Not the half marathons I had previously run. No, it would be the full thing—a whopping 26.2 miles. But I began to put a little bit of pressure on myself.

Knowing I now carried the label and identity of a *brain injury survivor* built a lot of pressure. It wasn't enough just to finish a race without walking or falling. Now, I wanted to compete at a higher level and live up to the expectations I thought others required of me (in addition to the expectations I placed on myself).

In 2015, I had a very audacious goal in mind: I was going to qualify for the Boston Marathon. Even more audacious of a goal: I was going to qualify in my hometown at the 2015 Pittsburgh Marathon, which was my first-ever full marathon. The qualification for the Boston Marathon for my age group in 2015 was to finish in under three hours and five minutes—but even then you were not guaranteed a spot. The lower your time was under 3:05, the better your chances to be selected to run the iconic race.

For a while during the 2015 Pittsburgh Marathon, I was on pace to actually qualify for the Boston Marathon. About nineteen miles in, I hit the proverbial wall (if you're a runner, you probably know what I'm talking about). The proverbial wall is the point in a race or a training run where you just can't move any faster. Your body is done—you want to lie down and just stop.

"I can't do this anymore, this is as good as it's going to get," I told myself. "You're a brain injury survivor, and you got almost twenty miles in. Great job!"

As I'm hitting the wall and my body is giving up, I happen to pass by ReMed, the facility where I had previously spent five days a week in brain rehabilitation as an outpatient. For 35 to 40 hours each week, I'd spend time retraining my brain through a variety of therapies. I was there from January 2014 into a major part of 2015. When I saw the building, I thought about the patients there who were fighting for their lives. These people were trying to regain function and control of their bodies, whether as inpatients or outpatients. By the grace of God, I was on the outside. *Some of the patients who I was with a year prior could still be in rehab,* I thought to myself. I had to finish this race!

At this point, my mental toughness kicked in. I realized I had to be a *leader of one* or suffer the consequences: *Leader of one, leader of many; if I can't lead one, I can't lead any.*

Being a *leader of one* means you're going through something that you haven't experienced before. You are going through the wilderness of life. Your adversity is your blessing—your trial might be what sets a trail for someone else.

A *leader of one* mentality means you have confidence and faith that the Lord will lead you. Just as He led the Israelites as they wandered in the desert for 40 years, you can have faith that the Lord will get you where you need to go. It's not always pleasant or easy, but when you've been in the trenches as a *leader of one,* you are prepared to be in the trenches for someone else, too. This can look like an encouraging word to a friend, supporting a loved one in prayer, or even attending your child's sporting event.

From Mile 19 to the finish line, I walked off and on. But I did that because I had to be the *leader of one* (a leader to myself) and finish the race. Although I was in my own metaphorical trench, I knew the Lord was walking with me every step of the race. That encouraging thought kept me going.

As I kept thinking back to the ReMed building, I also thought about Harold Squibbs, a friend of mine and fellow brain injury survivor, whom I met while at the rehab facility. I knew that Harold would be volunteering at the Pittsburgh Marathon. I'm not sure if I ever promised him directly that I would finish the race. But in my mind, I made a promise to a friend, and I was determined to keep it.

Harold wasn't a runner. But the race was his just as much as it was mine. Harold encouraged me leading up to race day and was excited for me to run. Harold was a big reason why I even finished the race.

The Monday after the 2015 Pittsburgh Marathon, I went into ReMed, the facility where I had my brain rehabilitation. I sat in the lobby waiting to give Harold my medal. Giving away my medals to other people (especially to those who have encouraged me or have been there for me) reminds me that the race is not about the destination, but rather all about the journey.

As I waited for Harold, there was a gentleman in a wheelchair nearby.

He noticed me sitting in my chair with the medal around my neck and said to me, "I'm going to run a marathon someday."

The man's caregiver standing next to him said something along the lines of, "It's not realistic for you to run." WOW! I hope he proved that person wrong.

For me, that was a God moment. I hope that the

gentleman in the wheelchair brushed off the negativity and continued to be a *leader of one* (a leader to himself) and received the encouragement he needed to keep pursuing his dream.

Harold's encouragement from race day motivated me to be a leader of one. His encouragement has always impacted so many others and during that moment, he motivated me to do the same thing moving forward.

"For the Spirit God gave us does not make us timid, but gives us power, love and self-discipline."

— 2 TIMOTHY 1:7

CHAPTER 3

Make It Personal, Don't Take It Personally

RACE: 2017 ERIE PRESQUE ISLE MARATHON;
RESULT: 3:11:51, MILE PACE: 7:19/MI

Take a moment and imagine the following scenario: The CEO of a major company is at a job site. He's got a ton of items on his mind. While at the job site, something goes wrong. So, he goes to the office and snaps at the secretary. She gets upset and takes out her frustration on her assistant. Then her assistant gets mad and takes it out on the intern. The frustration trickles down the line to everyone in the company.

What's happening? As the saying goes, everyone is "kicking the cat." Poor kitty!

I share this illustration to tell you this: when we *take something personally,* we often take the negative things people have said to us, and repeat them to ourselves. These comments affect our self-worth, confidence, and the core of who we are as human beings. *Taking things personally* can really take a toll on your mental health and emotional well-being.

But when you *make something personal,* you have *ownership.* Let me repeat that . . . If you make something personal, you have ownership. Therefore, you can control the situation instead of letting the situation control you. You can hold yourself accountable, take responsibility, and have a stake in the *outcomes* of whatever situation you're facing.

When you learn to *make it personal,* you realize life can be created or taken away with words. As 2 Timothy says, you have been given a spirit of self-control. Practicing self-control is the root of what it means to *make it personal.*

In 2017, I was running the most confident race I had competed in since I first started training eight weeks after my brain injury. It was here at the 2017 Erie Presque Isle Marathon I was running conservatively at a 7:07 mile pace for the first seventeen miles. I knew I needed to kick things into high gear at Mile 20 with a 7:05 mile pace to qualify for the Boston Marathon. So far, my plan was working—I was right where I needed to be.

NOTE: Read this part carefully! I had plans to qualify for the Boston Marathon: this was it! My plan was finally working. I always say, "If you want to tell God a joke, tell him your plans." What are you going to do and what is the conversation going to be with him

*when you don't get what you want to get and when you
want to get it?*

Just before Mile 18, my right shoelace felt loose.

"I know it's on," I thought. "I know my shoelace is loosening, but it's not a problem. I won't trip on it because I'm aware of it. Everything is good."

I kept running at my 7:07 mile pace.

At Mile 18, my shoelace somehow came undone. Not only did I trip over the shoelace, but it basically tangled itself into my left shoe. I went down like a ton of bricks. I fell and actually hit the side of my face. My legs were cut up, and I had a cut right above my left eyebrow. I definitely had a few choice words come to mind.

Then, I *took the fall too personally*.

"I'm done," I told myself. "I'm not going to qualify for the Boston Marathon. I fell down, and I can't do this anymore."

I thought maybe the fall only happened to me because I had a brain injury or a case of bad luck.

I took a moment and just sat in my self-pity. But then I remembered another friend of mine who had texted me the day before the race. He had gone through a ton of medical turmoil. The day before the race, he texted me saying he was proud of me and thanked me for encouraging him in his journey.

At that moment, *I made my race situation personal.*

Instead of feeling sorry for myself, I realized you

don't always get what you want (and when you want it, for that matter). I needed to drop that childish mentality! When we *take things personally*, we either quit or we "kick the cat." Neither of those are great outcomes. But when you *make a situation personal*, you choose what you create. You are responsible for your actions and the outcomes that arise. I had an opportunity to *pivot with purpose* and still make something of my situation at Mile 18. So I got up and I finished the race.

My pace slowed from 7:07 during the first seventeen miles to a 7:11 pace for miles eighteen to twenty-six. The funny thing is I ended up setting a PR (personal record) by finishing the race in three hours and eleven minutes. Ultimately, I was glad that I finished what I started. By *making the race personal* instead of *taking it personally*, I got to recreate the outcome for the last few miles of the race.

Additionally, I qualified for the Chicago Marathon. The qualifying time for that race was three hours and fifteen minutes, and my PR time at the Presque Isle Marathon qualified with four minutes to spare. I was totally surprised!

The last thing I'll say is mastering the art of *making it personal* helps build your character. God is writing your story, but you can take it an extra step and *make it personal* by working to craft the character you want to be by the end of your chapter. I say chapter because your story isn't over yet. You only need to focus on the character you want to be, and let God take care of the rest.

"Therefore everyone who hears these words of mine and puts them into practice is like a wise man who built his house on the rock."

— MATTHEW 7:24

CHAPTER 4

Wake Up to the Whisper of the Lord

RACE: 2021 JOEY FABUS 5K; RESULT: 18:59,
MILE PACE: 6:15/MI

Nowadays, everyone is so used to the rat race of waking up and getting the day started. We live in a world that is constantly on-the-go from morning till night, with little rest in between. We have families and work and after-school activities. There are errands to run and meals to prepare and friends to see. When are we supposed to rest?

Early on in my running career, especially after the first half marathon, I would wake up and run first thing in the morning. I started to get more serious about my goals, and as they grew, I thought I needed to put the work in before everybody else awoke. I would run before brain rehabilitation or anything else I had going on that day. I also would make time to do some personal development of my choice in order to help my brain heal. I figured I was starting my day out in the best possible way.

Did you know that 1% of your day is the equivalent to about fourteen minutes? In the grand scheme of daily life, fourteen minutes takes up almost a quarter of an hour (or 840 seconds). It's pretty minimal if you ask me.

During my recovery, I decided to change my morning routine to *wake up to the whisper of the Lord*. This concept means that you're going from powering down at night to then turning yourself on in the morning by waking up to God's voice. Rather than reaching for your phone, starting a workout, or making breakfast, you're taking time (maybe fourteen minutes or so) to listen to what the Lord is saying to you. By choosing to spend one percent of your day with God, you're setting yourself up for the best day ever. And if you practice *waking up to the whisper of the Lord* on a daily basis, the benefits will compound over time.

The world tries to dictate the conversation you have with yourself every time you turn on the news, check your email, or check the weather app. Most of the time, the world only has negative things to say. But when you *wake up to the whisper of the Lord*, you learn how to listen. You learn to hear the word of God and understand it a little bit clearer. You find encouragement for the day ahead. That time spent is better than anything you'll hear on the daily news cycle.

After my brain injury, I struggled to listen to understand, rather than listening to respond. I struggled to understand what someone was saying, because it felt way too fast (even if they were talking slowly or even at a normal pace). Plus, the second you begin listening, your brain starts to formulate a response. To practice conversation with others, I had to practice listening to the *whisper of the Lord*. This began by truly listening, without formulating any response at all.

What does the *whisper of the Lord* sound like? For me, it's the things I hear from the Lord in the quiet dark of the morning rather than the roaring words of the world. It's still dark when I get up, but I can hear birds chirping and other creatures buzzing and roaming about that I normally wouldn't hear. I would miss the opportunity to hear these beautiful noises if I had just got up and started moving and making my own noise. And we all miss this from time to time just for the chance to get out the door as quickly as we can.

You must give yourself time to listen to the Lord, which may take some practice. Stillness is a practice. I *wake up to the whisper of the Lord* sometimes at 4 a.m., sometimes at 4:30 a.m. Afterwards, I do my workout at 5:30 a.m. You may need to adjust your routine. If you're going to wake up earlier, whether fourteen minutes or longer, you need to create a pivot right there so you can go to bed earlier. That's where you determine your goals and understand where to *pivot with purpose.*

As I've gotten older, I know that I've gotten better because I *wake up to the whisper of the Lord.* I have come to realize there's nothing more important than starting my day by spending time with God. This can look differently depending on the season I am facing. Sometimes I will pray for others or I will journal. But mostly, I will read my Bible or a devotional. What is most amazing about this is sometimes I'll read something in my Bible and a verse or a passage will remind me of someone or something someone said; this makes me want to read a little deeper. This practice of reading scripture helps me focus and dive deeper into the words God shares with his people. It also sets me up for a successful day because my heart posture is one that's open and prepared to listen to whoever I speak with that day.

Don't get me wrong—you're still going to have days where you want to hit the snooze button or you'll want to just get up and go because there are so many things to do. But when you get your bearings straight . . . when you *wake up to the whisper of the Lord* and you just listen . . . it makes a real difference. Let me give you an example.

In 2021, I ran the Joey Fabus 5K, a local 5K in my neighborhood. This 5K hits close to home and is held every year in his memory. While in middle school, Joey died of an incurable, untreatable cancer. His cancer is called Diffuse Intrinsic Pontine Glioma (DIPG) and the current survival rate is 0%. Most children afflicted with this disease die within nine to twelve months of the initial diagnosis. Joey's family has been raising money for research since his passing in 2015.

The night before the race, I went to bed as a child of God.

"I am who I am," I thought.

I didn't think about the race, or my identity as a runner. I didn't wear my running gear to bed like I normally do before a race. I simply went to bed and knew I would *wake up to the whisper of the Lord* the next day.

On race day, I got to the destination and took my time to put on my running gear. I felt calm and immensely thankful for the opportunity to run and raise money to find a cure. It was a 5k that was way bigger than my running goals or running identity.

I started warming up and stretching.

As I approached the starting line, a random person looked at me, pointed a finger and said, "My money's on that guy."

That was the first race I've ever been at where something like that happened. But since I had *woken up to the whisper of the Lord*, I had no pressure and wasn't thinking about the race too much. I just showed up, warmed up, and someone randomly said that they thought I'd win the Joey Fabus 5K. Funnily enough, it was actually the first 5K that I ever won.

I leave you with this challenge: learn how to *wake up to the whisper of the Lord*. Even if this means you wake up fourteen minutes earlier. That 1% of waking up and listening to the Lord will set you up for success for the rest of your life. Or maybe you can take fourteen minutes sitting in the car before going to work . . .

just listen. Maybe it's taking those fourteen minutes right before walking in the door to work. The older we get, the more hats we wear. We are going so fast we don't usually know which hat we are wearing (spouse, friend, athlete, colleague, parent, etc.). Taking the time to be still and let God whisper to you allows you to be alert for the moments throughout the day when you have to switch hats, and believe me, you will. I believe you are worth that 1% daily, but do you?

"Am I now trying to win the approval of human beings, or of God? Or am I trying to please people? If I were still trying to please people, I would not be a servant of Christ."

— GALATIANS 1:10

CHAPTER 5
Think, Act, Try Again, Adjust

RACE: 2016 ERIE PRESQUE ISLE MARATHON;
RESULT: 3:41:25, MILE PACE: 8:27/MI

I've created a little formula that I believe will help you in your athletic pursuits and faith walk:

Think. Act. Try Again. Adjust.

Let's start with the first step: *Think*. The majority of people are pretty good thinkers. You likely have a great set of critical thinking skills, and you probably have thought about where you'd like your life to go. You've set some goals, you have big dreams, and you are full of ideas. And I'm guessing they are pretty great ideas.

Thinking is great. But what happens after that? Taking a thought and putting it into action is a totally different story. When you think and take action, you put something in motion. And an object in motion tends to stay in motion.

When you simply think about something, it doesn't

progress. Where does it go? A thought remains a thought until you put action behind it.

And this is what trips up the majority of the population. Most people don't take the time to back up their thoughts with actions, no matter how big or small those thoughts are.

God doesn't want us to remain stagnant. Instead, He calls us to the next step: *Act*. Remember when He called Moses to speak to the Israelites as they wandered in the wilderness? Remember Moses' reaction? He thought and thought. He worried and told God that he wasn't a speaker. But God called Moses to act anyway. In faith and with the help of his brother Aaron, Moses listened to the Lord and responded by taking action.

There's a quote that says, "If you give me four hours to cut down a tree, I'll spend three hours sharpening my ax." Some people spend all their time sharpening their ax but never use it to act. Don't be that person.

One important part about brain injury survivors is that every individual's brain injury is unique. You can't compare your recovery to someone else's recovery. You can't expect to make progress without having to *Try Again* and *Adjust* your recovery plan.

The same is true for running. I've made so much progress in my races and training because I decided I am only in competition with myself. As Jim Rohn says, "Work harder on yourself than you do on your job." I stay in my lane, avoid distractions, and focus on training harder by moving faster than I did before. By trying again and making adjustments, I compete with myself in a healthy way, while also creating repetition. Over time, repetition becomes a habit.

If you *Think, Act, Try Again,* and *Adjust,* you're learning how to live in a state of progress over perfection (we'll talk about this a few chapters from now). When you follow this formula, you will absolutely start to see results because you are growing and learning. If you don't follow the steps, you'll always live in a state of procrastination. You'll never take the first step, you'll never make a mistake, and you'll never win or lose . . . and that would be pretty sad, because I want to see you progress.

In 2016, I ran the Erie Presque Isle Marathon in three hours, forty-one minutes, and twenty-five seconds. That's about an 8:27 mile finish. In 2017, I ran the race again—same distance, but a year apart. However, my final time was three hours, eleven minutes and fifty-one seconds. My mile pace was 7:19. I went from an 8:27 mile pace in 2016 to a 7:18 mile pace in 2017. How?

Think. I decided to run the 2017 Erie Presque Isle Marathon.

Act. I took action and began training for the 2017 Erie Presque Isle Marathon.

Try Again. I kept training. I worked hard and focused on my goals. I kept going.

Adjust. I made some adjustments both physically and mentally. If something didn't work, I tried again or looked for a better solution.

And then what happened after that? I repeated this process over and over until it came time to race in the 2017 Erie Presque Isle Marathon. By the way, this process is not for the faint of heart. It is hard work. I don't want you to get the wrong idea. Athletic training of any kind is not easy.

But guess what? Faith isn't easy either. Faith requires hard work and training, too. And just how no one's race is the same, no one's faith is the same. My faith is different from yours, and that's perfectly fine. My faith journey looks different from yours, and that's okay, too. The race set before me might be different from the race set before you. Maybe we should all focus on our personal faith journeys with as much zeal as we place on our personal records.

And because we recognize that faith doesn't always come so easily and understand that Jesus died and sacrificed His life for us, it's time to put in the work. The Lord is light, and once you know the light, you have to make a choice. Is it worth the hard work, training, and sacrifice to grow your faith and share the light with others? Absolutely.

Progress doesn't happen overnight. You have to put

in the work. In time, it gets easier as you get used to repetition and begin to build good habits. Speaking of habits, use each opportunity to *Think, Act, Try Again, and Adjust*. Not only will this habit end up supporting your goals and dreams, but it will also build up your faith.

"I long to see you so that I may impart to you some spiritual gift to make you strong—that is, that you and I may be mutually encouraged by each other's faith."

— ROMANS 1:11-12

CHAPTER 6
Be Encouraged Every Day

RACE: 2022 JOEY FABUS 5K; RESULT 20:21,
MILE PACE: 6:30/MI

Have you ever heard the phrase, "Excitement can't be caught, but it can be taught"?

After my brain injury, I learned what this phrase meant. It means that anyone can learn to get excited. Maybe you are a runner and get excited after a really great training run. Or maybe you are the parent of an athlete and get really excited when your son or daughter does well by making a big play during their sporting event.

Excitement can't be caught, but it can be taught.

I believe that the same rule applies for encouragement. We can't catch encouragement, but we can learn how to encourage ourselves and others. We can teach ourselves to be encouraged every day.

There are days when we wake up on the right side of the bed and feel encouraged. But the majority of the time we wake up, we aren't immediately encouraged. That's because 80% of the conversations we have in this life are internal—you know—the ones we have with ourselves. And often, we don't think to encourage ourselves. But, with practice, you and I can both learn to speak positively to ourselves and others.

To encourage others is to encourage ourselves. If you encourage others, they are likely going to do or say something that will encourage you later. Sometimes, others will encourage you and in the moment, you won't even know it until you reflect back. So, aim to encourage at least one person every day. It may take days, weeks, months, or years for them to appreciate your intention, but you know the ripple effect it can establish.

Following this practice is the same thing as waking up to the whisper of the Lord. Remember that when you wake up to God's whisper, you hear the words that the Lord is whispering with more clarity. When you practice, you begin to be able to hear Him in the middle of your day or week, too. If you encourage someone, they will also wake up to encouragement.

The other day, my two-year-old and her older sister were playing outside. My two-year-old would not listen and go inside. Now, of my two little girls, I believe she's going to be a runner. Her legs are like the Road Runner—fast, furious, and out of control. She wears out her older sister, but she just loves to run. As I try to corral her inside, she asks, "Daddy, can I chase you?"

She didn't understand, but her question meant so much. It encouraged me.

I shouldn't be alive for so many reasons (the brain injury being the most obvious reason). And it's a miracle that I can walk, or even run and compete in marathons in that respect.

I said, "Yes!"

Hearing my little girl ask if she can chase me is one of the most encouraging things I have ever heard.

Encouragement doesn't always have to be a grand gesture. Sometimes, encouragement is a simple hello, or offering someone a quarter so they can use a shopping cart at Aldi. Side note: If you haven't shopped there, you're missing out! I encourage you to stop by and maybe offer a quarter to someone who needs it.

On other days, encouragement is a totally different beast.

In 2022, I ran the Joey Fabus 5K. I'd run it the previous year and the course setup was the same. The race is held around Bethel Park Middle School (formerly known as Independence Middle School), and it's an extremely hilly course. The course is hilly in part due to Pittsburgh being hilly as is, but also because there are so many hills around the Bethel Park campus.

The funny thing about all this is that back in 2021, the Joey Fabus 5K became the first 5K I ever won. But it doesn't stop there. There was a kid who also ran the 5K but didn't officially enter the race and didn't have a registered race chip. Technically, this kid crossed the line before I did, but it didn't count because he wasn't officially registered as a participant. When he crossed the finish line sans chip, it set off a series of technical errors. My winning time wasn't marked. By the time I crossed, the recording system was all out of whack. The race directors apologized and admitted the mistake, but it didn't matter. I didn't let it get me down. As runners we get so caught up in the weeds of results. I have been there, and sometimes it's still a battle. Knowing my effort in this win is what mattered. The race was about raising money and supporting a grieving family. My time or finish was a tiny part of the whole picture.

The week before the 2022 Joey Fabus 5K, I disqualified myself after ten miles in the 2022 Erie Marathon. But I moved forward and focused on the 5K. I felt good. I felt ready to compete again. Heck, I was really looking forward to it.

Then, I recognized the kid from the previous year who had technically crossed the finish line before me. He had entered and registered this time around. I knew he would be my only competition for the entire race, and I made a mental note to pass him early.

When the race starts, this kid bolts out front—like he was shot out of a cannon. Another guy next to him does the same thing. They go out flying at a blazing speed, and I'm behind both of them. But I remembered this course has hills—lots of uphills and only two downhills. The first downhill starts the course. The second downhill is almost at the finish line.

I know that I can catch these guys on the hills, or at

least the kid who beat me in 2021. Within the first tenth of a mile, we go down a hill, around a neighborhood, and then back uphill past the school.

The kid that beat me last year stopped coming back uphill after that first downhill. He had started way too fast. He was hunched over. When I passed him, I gave him a pat on the back, and some encouragement. I didn't stop—we were competing, after all—but I knew he was low on energy and that a little bit of encouragement would lift him up. So, I encouraged him.

At this point, I'm in second place, and the other guy is still blazing pretty fast. We go up around the school, then back on a flat, then up another hill, and I start catching this guy. On the second hill of the race, the elevation is pretty hard. I could tell this hill was too much for him on this day.

That's when it dawned on me: Hills don't kill. Cancer does.

We all have hills in life. Or we see an obstacle and we think it's going to kill us. Honestly, we humans are pretty dramatic.

I get up to this guy and pat him on the back. But this time, I yell out, "Hills don't kill, cancer does!" I got emotional because I thought about the "hill" that Joey Famus' family was forced to climb. They lost a son to incurable childhood cancer. As that is not enough, they choose to keep climbing to find a cure for other kids and families.

And I keep yelling that statement because it's true.

But I also kept shouting that phrase because I think I was not only encouraging others, but also myself.

When I get to the top of the hill, I'm all by myself. I'd accidentally gone the wrong way and had gotten way off course. By the time I get turned around, the guy who I had passed is now back and up this hill, too.

He sees me. But instead of taking off, knowing that he would be ahead of me, this guy slowed down and waited for me to catch up.

When I get back to him, he says, "Thank you so much. I wouldn't have finished this race if you didn't encourage me."

I said, "Let's go, let's finish this strong." So we went back down the hill.

As we go back down, we start passing other runners who are also competing in this race. They're mostly athletes who are in good shape, but every single one is struggling with the hill.

I start shouting as loudly as I can, "Hills don't kill, cancer does!"

I'm flying down the hill now as I near the final straightaway—I'm blazing. I notice that the pace car, or the car that keeps pace with the lead runner, isn't moving yet. I don't think the pace car was expecting any runners so soon.

It starts up, eventually, and now all I see is the last straightaway. It was maybe a quarter of a mile. This whole time, I believe I'm by myself. It's just between me and the pace car, which was a surreal feeling in itself. It felt like watching the elite runner or the elite pack bunched together just behind the pace car in the New York City Marathon, or any other Abbott World Major Marathons that I've watched over the years.

Right before the finish line, there are two quick turns before you end up back in the school parking lot. The turns slow you down a lot—going from a straight-away into a sharp left and then a sharp right just before the finish line. As I went to step across the finish line, the guy who was on the hill inched past me.

His hands were on his knees as soon as the race was over. I could tell he was beat. I was tired as well.

He goes, "I'm so sorry I won the race. You deserve that race."

I told him he did good, that he gave it everything he had and beat me.

We ended up running three miles together to cool down. We jogged and talked. We encouraged each other and we encouraged ourselves.

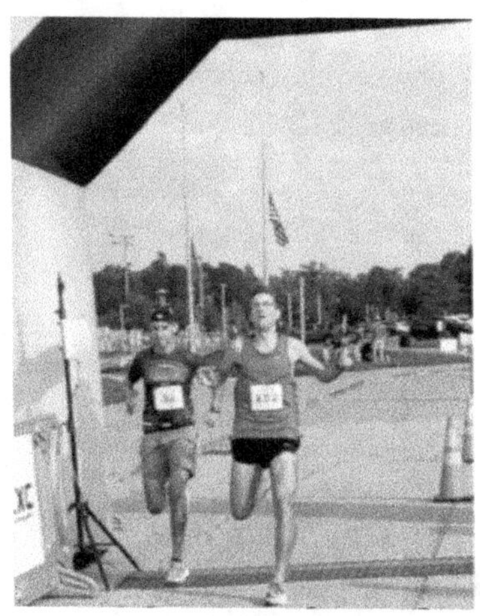

2022 Joey Fabus 5k finish line.

PART TWO
Leaning Forward

"The Word became flesh and made his dwelling among us. We have seen his glory, the glory of the one and only Son, who came from the Father, full of grace and truth."

— JOHN 1:14

CHAPTER 7

Your Personal Narrative

As humans, we are innately drawn to the idea of story. We learn in school that every story has a beginning, a middle, and an end. Every great story includes a hero who is on a path to overcome an obstacle or save a heroine. The heroes often learn more about themselves along the way. Stories help us connect with others, teach us lessons, and remind us of what we have overcome.

Your story is unique. It's completely yours, and no one else in the world has a story quite like yours.

We often ask each other, "What's your story?"

But I'm going to challenge you to ask yourself some different questions:

- What's the narrative I hear from others?
- What's the personal narrative I tell myself?
- What does God's word say?

- Do I know my personal narrative?

Most people are doing the same thing over and over again. They either listen to the story they tell themselves (whether accurate or not), or they listen to the story others are telling about them.

One secret I've learned over the years is that you have to avoid the pitfalls of others. Don't take what others say personally. There's a chance they are taking their emotions out on you or simply projecting. If you're not aware of their narrative, it can become yours. You have to be able to take yourself out of the situation and observe as a bystander. Hold on to the narrative you've created—one with Christ at the center.

As a Christian, your personal narrative is the most important tool in your arsenal. You obviously play a role in your story. Others can play a role in your story, too. But the biggest part of your story is actually *God's story*. In His word, you discover what He says about you—how He loved you so much that He sent His only son to die for you. He rose to life three days later to show He overcame death on your behalf.

When you have a personal narrative centered in Christ, you can identify who you are and the person you are going to be. Our God is the same yesterday, today, and tomorrow. When you retrospectively look at your personal narrative through the years, it's easier to see how God has been there the whole time. You can see how your faith has grown over months and years through all of the various trials life brings you through.

For a while, my personal narrative was that I didn't invite God into my story. Prior to my brain injury, my personal narrative was that I would be in the NBA as a means to an end—to make money to support my mom. But I didn't make room for God to be a part of that conversation. I had placed so much pressure on myself to perform for a solid 20 years of my life, and the pressure to perform didn't leave me when it came to running. Once God's story became my story, I saw a huge shift.

My personal narrative really shaped itself and grew during the 2022 Pittsburgh Marathon. In that race, I hit my current marathon personal record (PR) for three hours and seven minutes. You could see my character through running. You could see my growth over time. When you start to understand your personal narrative, your relationships start to change. When you change your perception, you change your reality. When you know your personal narrative (like it or not), you can start to implement those big changes in your life.

Before the 2022 Pittsburgh Marathon, my best marathon time was three hours and eleven minutes, which I hit during the 2017 Erie Presque Isle Marathon. But I made a few changes to my personal narrative. First, I switched over to a new coach in 2021. My current coach who I was connected with, Jimmy Stevens, played a huge role in my success and results of 2022. Sometimes it takes one person to show up in your life and teach you the importance of letting God have the final say. Because of our relationship, my faith has grown, and the pressure to perform has weakened. I had so much confidence in the 2022 marathon because I learned the impact of who I am and allowed my personal narrative to change.

When I got to the starting line at the 2022 Pittsburgh Marathon, Coach Jimmy said, "Listen, I know you're not used to this, but I want you to fuel with a gel every 5k." I followed his instructions, and I ended up with my PR. I shaved twenty-one minutes off from my previous time of three hours and twenty-six minutes. The 2022 Pittsburgh Marathon was also a four-minute personal best finish from my three hours, eleven minute time in the 2017 Erie Presque Isle Marathon. It was largely due to Coach Jimmy's expertise and the change in my personal narrative. The best thing about all of this is that I love my personal narrative more now than I ever had before.

If you don't love your personal narrative, you have the power to change it. If you don't believe me, think about your personal narrative as it is today. Sit down and ask yourself, "What's my story?" "What am I telling myself?" Dig into God's word and learn what He says about you. It's fine to want to change, but first you have to understand the current narrative you speak over yourself. You cannot change what you are not aware of. Are you aware of the truths (accurate or not) you tell yourself? That is your current narrative.

Change your perception, and then change your reality.

NOTE: Let me share with you the progress I have made in the Pittsburgh Full Marathon. I am sharing this with you to PRESS upon you — not impress you. Time management is self-management. If you can manage yourself, then you can manage your time and become more efficient at just about anything. The distance of 26.2 miles is the same for each race, but my finishing time has changed. My mindset has changed because my God has changed me.

- *2015 Pittsburgh Marathon: Finish 5:49:01 at 13:09/mi*
- *2016 Pittsburgh Marathon: Finish 4:05:03 at 9:21/mi*
- *2018 Pittsburgh Marathon: Finish 3:26:04 at 7:51/mi*
- *2022 Pittsburgh Marathon: Finish at 3:07:20 at 7:09/mi (I went to the stall twice and it cost me a Boston Qualify Time. But that's okay!)*
- *2023 Pittsburgh Marathon: 3:18:14 at 7:33/mi (This is an hour off of the Olympic Qualify Standard time of 2:18:00 cut off. KEEP GOING!!! I'll show up until I can't.)*

"Jesus said, 'Father, forgive them, for they do not know not what they are doing.' And they divided up his clothes by casting lots."

— LUKE 23:34

CHAPTER 8
Prayer Over Pain

RACE: 2021 BUFFALO CREEK HALF
MARATHON; RESULT: 1:25:22, MILE PACE
6:31/MI

A really good friend of mine, Matt Scoletti, used to say, "Embrace the suck." When you embrace the suck, you're basically telling your mind to be on guard. Something is coming, and it's going to get you. Tighten up, batten down the hatches, and get ready for whatever obstacle is on its way.

Now he says, "Seek the suck." Why the switch?

Well, the change follows a few of the principles we've already covered in this book. First, we already know pain is not pleasant. When you make it personal and seek the suck, you get to own the pain that is inevitably coming. Yes, it's going to hurt, but the more times you overcome it, the less it will hurt. You won't be caught off guard by just letting the suck find you. *Think, act, try again,* and *adjust.* You can make adjustments along the way and, eventually, you'll get over the hurdle.

Being a Christian means fighting for faith, enduring suffering, obeying the Lord, and making sacrifices. The prayer part of *prayer over pain* means to focus on praying for yourself, your family, and the world. Jesus endured the ultimate pain and sacrifice when He died on the cross. When you pray, you know there will be pain in this lifetime. When you pray despite the pain, you're acknowledging the Lord is sovereign in the midst of that pain.

My word of the year for 2023 is "furnace." I'm going into the furnace, which is extremely painful, but I know that God will be with me every step of the way.

I have spent so many of my marathons with new runners who are scared of the proverbial wall. Even if they've completed marathons in the past, they don't want to run into the wall or even talk about it. They know it's painful. But I know something they don't; the pain doesn't last as long as we often convince ourselves and I'm ultimately able to overcome the pain quicker because of prayer. When you pray, you can accept those hardships, and then you can grow.

In 2021, I ran the Buffalo Creek Half Marathon. I'd been going to physical therapy for a little while for help alleviating some minor issues. I don't remember which mile I was on. But, at one point, I knew I was going to hit the wall in the half marathon based on the issues I'd been dealing with. I knew the pain was coming, and I prayed about it. I was prepared for the pain.

Ironically, my right shoelace came loose after mile nine or ten of a 13.12-mile race. I knew I had to tie the lace, so I bent down and tied it.

This was a perfect example that *if you don't take care of the little things now, they will become big and take care of you.* Flashback to the Erie Half Marathon when I chose not to tie my shoelace because I didn't think I had time to do so. I was worried I would lose my pace to qualify for the Boston Marathon. But in reality, not taking the time to tie it caused me to trip.

Stop tripping over quarters in your life to pick up a dollar bill! Are you tripping over little things in your life? Then take your time and tie up the loose ends.

In this Buffalo Creek Half Marathon, I bent down to tie it. It made me stop in my tracks and think, "Man, this really hurts." I felt the pain in my right calf and right hamstring.

I almost let it affect me and the rest of the race. We, as humans, tend to be dramatic.

Instead, I got right back up. My faith was growing, even though I knew the wall was coming and the pain would soon follow.

Experts say if you stop in the middle of a marathon, you won't be able to start back up. It's going to hurt even more when you get going again. There was pain, but I got right back up. I finished the race three minutes faster than the year before. When you have *prayer over pain*, you're prepared. You know the pain is coming, but you keep going anyway. Reframe your mindset on pain and know God is with you each step of the race. Expect pain, but pray anyway. You'll be thankful you did and you will feel accomplished when, by His grace, you make it to the other side.

"For Christ's sake, I delight in weaknesses, in insults, in hardships, in persecutions, in difficulties. For when I am weak, then I am strong."

— 2 CORINTHIANS 12:10

CHAPTER 9
Pay Attention to the Tension

RACE: 2023 PITTSBURGH MARATHON;
RESULT: 3:18:14, MILE PACE 7:33/MI

I've learned over time that tension is one of the most important aspects of being an athlete.

Tension works on three levels. There's physical tension. An example of this would be when you pull a hamstring and have to rest easy for a few days. Then there's mental tension. Maybe this could be a time when you're going back and forth on different strategies to reach a goal. You are caught between wanting to decrease your average mile pace, but also doubting if you would be able to do so. And lastly, let's not forget about emotional tension. You are faced with the bittersweet moment of finishing a race. You are ecstatic about your race outcome, but also a little sad that it is over. This means it's time to start training for the next marathon.

The key to dealing with any type of tension is that you first need to recognize it. This is absolutely essential. Knowing how to listen for the tension in your life is vital for your emotional, physical, social and mental health. Athletes, especially young athletes, need to know tension plays a role in everything. For years, I used running as an escape, or distraction so I could avoid the tension of my brain injury. I've finally learned this about myself as I've gotten older. But I hope you can learn to recognize this truth now at whatever stage you're at in your life, whether applicable to your athletic career or personal endeavors.

Tension can be both good and bad. Sometimes it can signal an imbalance in the body. Other times, it's a tug at your heart.

Tension is also a choice.

It creates awareness. Awareness allows you to make a decision, which can lead to growth, if you let it. You have the ability to stay in your comfort zone, or leave it. You can prioritize tension or ignore it. But ultimately, the choice is up to you.

One day while running errands, I heard a great analogy about tension. In the podcast I was listening to, Anthony Stanley said if you don't take care of your demons (which is tension) they will live in the basement of your soul and lift weights. If you don't take care of the tension when you feel it, a small issue can easily become bigger. You could have possibly avoided the bigger issue had you addressed the initial tension.

Most of us tend to avoid tension. We choose to ignore it or pretend it's not there, thinking it will go away on its own. But it doesn't work like that. Tension tells you what your strengths and weaknesses are. It teaches you how to pivot. When you're aware of what's going on, you can connect the dots. Tension teaches you what areas you need to grow toward. Tension also teaches you what areas you need to make strides toward in order to make progress (more on progress later). When we have strengths in our life, we tend to depend on those strengths to a point it leads to overcompensation. As a result, we experience a lack of growth.

Let me go on a really quick tangent. Going into the 2023 playoffs, the Golden State Warriors were the defending champions. In fact, if you follow them, they have become a dynasty. They have a superstar in Steph Curry. They have won titles in 2015, 2017, 2018, and 2022 because they played to their strengths better than any other team. They also made the best pivots I had ever seen a team make. However, one point to note is that in 2023, they were knocked out of the playoffs, and deservedly so, by Lebron James with the Los Angeles Lakers.

What happened?

The Golden State Warriors' weaknesses finally caught up to them. Strengths are great, but they aren't foolproof. Now, let's get back to your regularly scheduled programming, ha!

With runners (I am speaking from personal experience here) we have a tendency to train and hurt ourselves by not training properly. I like to call this the concept of a nick turning into a knack. Most runners decide to take shortcuts in their training because they don't have time for stretching. When I recently brought this up with my physical therapist, he ironically said *he doesn't even stretch*. Isn't it funny that a physical trainer whose job it is to tell patients to stretch won't do it himself?

Runners avoid the tension they feel because they want to put in the miles they know they need to aim toward. But if you avoid tension rather than prioritize it, the small nick becomes a bigger knack. And that knack left untreated can turn into a race day blow-up. Trust me, I've experienced it firsthand and seen it happen to plenty of others.

Unfortunately, this happened to a friend of mine the weekend I'm writing this. He ended up going into the marathon race with an injury, which led to utter disappointment. While he shifted his goal to just finishing the race, I could tell he was deflated. The problem was that he was competing really hard in the weeks leading up to the marathon. This caused the injury during the race that truly mattered. Maybe things would have gone differently if he had focused on the tension.

A few questions I would suggest you stop and ask yourself now are:

- What are my goals?
- What is an example of some tension (good or bad) that is up against my goals?

I'll never forget the physical tension I experienced in ninth grade. We still had the big analog clocks in the hallways, and as I was walking to class, I looked down the hall and realized I didn't have my assignment completed. As I walked and glanced up at the clock, I realized I was having a hard time seeing it as well as I normally could. It was blurry, which was interesting. But I didn't notice any pain! In my mind, I thought, *"Brilliant! When I get to class, I'll just tell my English teacher that I'm having trouble seeing out of my left eye, and I'll use this to my advantage. Maybe it'll give me more time to complete the assignment I didn't do."* But it was true—I was having difficulty reading the clock in the hallway. I paid attention to this seemingly small tension in my world. My eye didn't hurt, so that was good.

When I told my English teacher about my vision, she sent me to the nurse. I told her what was going on. I didn't know it then, but I was experiencing floaters in my eyes. The school nurse paid more attention to the tension than I did, and she made some phone calls. I felt bad for bringing up the blurry vision in the first place.

My mom and I ended up going to the Eye and Ear Institute in Pittsburgh. I was frustrated; I felt like we were wasting our time. But then I began feeling guilty. A new doctor examined my eyes. He knew my history and had reviewed everything. After the exam, he asked me straight up if I ever had retinal necrosis in my left eye.

"No," I said.

"Well, you do now," he replied.

His response hit me like a ton of bricks. I'd gone from trying to get out of completing a homework assignment to having a serious virus attacking my good eye—my only seeing eye.

But because I paid attention to the tension, and the teacher and the nurse had as well, it saved my vision. Retinal necrosis starts as a visual change, but no pain exists. However, in the span of 24 hours, the pain becomes excruciating, and it looks quite similar to pink eye (conjunctivitis). When the pain comes, it can cause the retina to detach. If left untreated, this can cause permanent loss of vision. It is a very painful and fast-acting virus.

This same thing happened again sixteen years later. In 2018, I had similar symptoms. Just as before, I paid attention to the tension, and again, my vision was saved. As soon as I felt the tension the second time around, I acted in urgency and got it looked at. I remember how quickly my vision was going in my left eye. Just before my vision really went away, I watched the 1999 Disney cartoon, *Tarzan*. I had to sit right in front of the television. After that day, I was legally blind and stayed home alone for roughly three weeks, while my wife went to work and had to take our daughter to my in-laws every day. I couldn't be with her during the day—I couldn't see. The doctors were able to get the virus under control, and my vision would eventually be restored. I had to rely on family and friends to drive me places and bring me food.

Thank the Lord that when I lost my vision—both when I was sixteen and later in 2018—that I paid attention to the physical tension. The vision was restored in my left eye both times, but unfortunately, I have not been able to see out of my right eye since I was thirteen.

If I can survive the things I have survived, then I know I can put myself out there to train to become an elite runner. Why not? If I fail, that's fine. Failure doesn't define me, that's what my Father does.

Another detail about tension is that you have to understand tension in order to be able to play with it. The process works best by living in the effort, and not the results.

In May 2023, I ran the Pittsburgh Marathon. Prior to the race, I was feeling really good. The mileage had been great, training had gone really well, and I was genuinely excited for race day. The week before the race, I was playing with my girls. Using a piece of chalk, I wrote my goal time of two hours and forty-five minutes for the race in chalk on our stone driveway. *"Goals in stone, plans in sand,"* I thought. I was feeling really confident.

However, on race day, I created unnecessary mental tension because I didn't follow my own rules. I took the race too personally. I let my fear of success taking the praise away from God get the best of me. I didn't live in the effort. Rather, I put the results *before* the effort, and it cost me.

My coach, Jimmy, drove all night and showed up to my house at 4 a.m. on zero sleep. He went down to the race with me, helped me warm up, took care of the details before the race, and took care of me before the race. He even paced me on and off during the race. He jumped all over the course, which I honestly don't know how he managed to do that, or how he even got ahead of me. But somehow, he did, and he pushed me. It was amazing.

During the race, Coach Jimmy knew what my pace should be right out of the gate. We wanted a pace of 6:40 per mile, and we'd work from there. We knew what my marks were . . . all that important stuff. And he pushed me. But I already created mental tension days prior, which I really didn't need on my plate. About thirteen miles in, I was predicting a three-hour finish. But by Mile 18, and right before I hit the wall at Mile 20, that pace and the results drastically changed. I started at a 7:02 pace, and kept it up halfway through the race. But by the last 10K, my average mile time had dropped to 7:31. I finished the race in three hours and eighteen minutes.

At first, I wasn't happy about the outcome. I was in pain, I felt horrible, and my performance wasn't ideal. But then I realized that twelve years ago, I had just run my first half marathon after a traumatic brain injury nearly ended my life, and I should have ended it to be frank. I ran that in two hours and ten minutes. Then I kept running and improving and watching the tension. And here, twelve years later, my full marathon race is way faster than the first half marathon I ever did. It's also better than my first full marathon race, which was five hours and forty-nine minutes during the 2015 Pittsburgh Marathon.

After the race, I went home and hugged my kids. I hung out with Coach Jimmy. I counted all my blessings. I enjoyed the rest of the weekend with my family.

Tension teaches you that you have to *live in the effort*. You have to deal with it. You have to run with effort every mile of a marathon. You have to have confidence. But you must also realize that you can't run the goal in the first mile. You have to take things one step, one mile, and one minute at a time.

One hindsight note about that race: learn to live with standards rather than expectations.

If you can live in the effort, you will organically create standards over time. And you will be able to handle and become more aware of the tension in your life.

Understand that tension can become different things and mean different things in your life. Tension can be toxic and lead to guilt and shame. It can also cause action and be a strength. You can either use tension in your life, or the tension will use you. Stop avoiding tension in your life—recognize it and decide what you are going to do with it.

Pay close attention to the tension in your life. What is it telling you? How will you respond?

"Listen to my prayer, O God, do not ignore my plea; hear me and answer me. My thoughts trouble me and I am distraught."

— PSALM 55:1-2

CHAPTER 10
Change Your Perception

RACE: 2019 PHILADELPHIA HALF MARATHON;
RESULT: 1:25:51, MILE PACE 6:33/MI

T he dictionary defines perception as "the state of being or process of becoming aware of something through the senses."

Perception is a big deal. You deal with how you are perceived especially as an athlete and even more so as a people of God. As Christians, we balance the perceptions of others daily. Some of these are kind, and others can often be unpleasant. But thankfully, the only perception that really matters is how God perceives us. The Lord perceives us as pure and holy thanks to His son, Jesus Christ's life, death, and resurrection. What a beautiful and precious gift!

Perception is also an important part of our mental health. Besides God's perception of who we are, we also have perceptions of ourselves or certain ways we observe our lives. Yet many people don't realize they have the power to *change* their perception.

How?

I'll let you in on a little secret. The biggest way to change your perception is by initiating action to change your mindset. You act first, because it then sets off a chain reaction. Once an action is taken, you have a new experience that you get to add to your personal narrative. You can *think, act, adjust,* and *try again* (like we talked about earlier).

You must also understand if you change your *perception*, you can also change your *reality*. But the *will to succeed* stems from the *will to change*. You can change your perception by sitting with your personal narrative or experiences, and reflecting on them.

If I ask someone what creature they fear the most in the ocean, the answer is likely going to be a shark. It makes sense, and I don't blame them. If you have a fear of sharks, you'd logically want to avoid swimming in the ocean.

But what if I took a shark out of water and put it on land? Do you think someone is going to still fear a shark on land? The answer is probably not. So what happened?

We changed your perception. When you change your *perception*, you can also change your *reality*.

Here's another example from Damon West, author of *Be the Coffee Bean*. At Jon Gordon's online Positive Summit in 2023, Damon explained how we're stuck in rush hour traffic many days of our lives. But he also asks readers why, on some days, the rush hour traffic just drives you bonkers. You're frustrated and you honk your horn. Then the very next day, you're still in rush hour traffic, but this time it doesn't bother you even in the slightest. What changed?

You did. Your *perception* about the situation changed. Your *mindset* changed.

The 2019 Philadelphia Half Marathon is a great example of how I changed my perception in order to change my reality. Heading into the Philadelphia Half Marathon, I was recovering from a summer of disappointment I faced as a result of my performance in the 2019 Erie Presque Isle Half Marathon. Before the Erie race, I'd over-hydrated all week because the weather predictions made it clear that the July race would be a warm one. My perception going into the half marathon was (and truly, my reality was) *it's going to be so hot*. I was so worried about the weather. The last thing any runner wants in a race is to be under-hydrated, cramping, and dealing with other ailments. I was so worried about everyone else's narratives, the narrative of the weather for the week, and narrative of the weather on race day. And I allowed those narratives to change my narrative.

I ended up not enjoying the race for multiple reasons. My results weren't what I had hoped for, and my performance ultimately suffered. I overcompensated by thinking about the weather instead of focusing on the race. On race day, I pivoted too much, thinking I couldn't handle the summer heat. To make a long story short, the last mile of the Erie Half Marathon ended up being my fastest.

I want you to understand that for several years after sustaining my brain injury, I was "injured." My perception truly didn't align with my reality. On May 5, 2013, I drove to downtown Pittsburgh and parked. I needed to get my Pittsburgh Marathon race packet at the Expo and parked within blocks of the building.

"This will be a quick in and out," I had thought.

In reality, it took me four hours to get into the building because I kept getting lost in the four-block radius of the David Lawrence Convention Center, which isn't a small building by any means. This was my first personal experience where I realized the significance of my brain injury. I was alone, because I thought I could accomplish the task of getting to the Expo on my own. It was the weirdest and most uncomfortable feeling of my life. I think many people (and especially brain injury survivors) can relate. You know where you are, but yet you don't. Reflecting on this day, it was like the Israelites walking for forty years on a trip that should have taken them forty days. Believe it or not, my worst days have become my best days because my worst days are when I know God was with me.

In 2015, I repeated the drive downtown to the race expo. I was feeling confident I could get in and out of the race Expo that day. However, some doubt was sneaking in because my perception was based on my previous experience of getting lost for four hours while I was picking up my race packet a couple of years before. This time though, I walked into the Expo with perfect efficiency and awareness of where I was. It was a huge win. Coming out and going back to my car did end up taking a little bit longer, because my memory was a bit fuzzy on where I had parked. My total time spent getting my race packet that year was only two hours. I had cut my race expo experience in half—a huge, exciting win!

Going into the 2019 Philadelphia Half Marathon, I knew my perception needed to change yet again. But to do this, I'd have to start taking action. And taking action often requires us to leave our comfort zone behind. I know you've heard plenty of phrases about the importance of getting out of your comfort zone. Let's be real and admit that getting out of our comfort zones sucks. It's not easy, and very few people actually enjoy doing it.

Let me share my new perception of race weekend. I took my perception and reality to a whole new level. I drove four hours from Pittsburgh to Philadelphia on my own. Being in the moment helped relieve some tension I typically experience on race day. I relaxed and just let things fly.

I got up the morning of the race and hopped on the bus. Along the way, I kept reassuring myself and reminding myself that perception is reality. Change your perception, and you can change your reality. Getting to the starting line, putting on a positive perspective, and having the confidence that I could do this helped put that mindset into action. I wasn't worried about trying to stay hydrated. I wasn't worried about the weather. I was living in the moment. I could have fixated on the chill in the air, but I didn't. I was focused solely on the race. I was excited, I was dressed properly, and I was ready to go. I got to the starting line feeling so relieved!

I ended up completing the 2019 Philadelphia Half Marathon with a new personal record after running a marathon just four months prior. On July 21, 2019, I finished the Erie Presque Isle Marathon in one hour, thirty-six minutes, and thirteen seconds. On November 24, 2019, I finished the Philadelphia Half Marathon with a time of one hour, twenty-five minutes, and fifty-one seconds.

What caused the change? My perception. I didn't *like what I was seeing*, so I took action, which caused a change in my perception. But more importantly, I didn't like *how I was feeling*. Are you tired of feeling tired, or are you tired of hiding your feelings? A word of caution: our feelings drive our actions and our perceptions. But feelings aren't facts. Let me repeat that: feelings aren't facts.

I'm blessed to have gone from once being lost to now being found, all thanks to the grace of God. Each race, and each year, my perception and reality transform. My faith continues to grow, and the pressure to perform drops significantly. I still have plenty of room to grow.

The Philadelphia Half Marathon showed me what I was truly capable of. It exhibited that I was only scratching the surface of possibility. That race also revealed a need to me. I should consistently pay attention to my own perception, because perception informs reality, after all. For better or worse, when you change one, you can also change the other.

Sometimes taking action can be scary. For things in your life to be comfortable or conventional, they must first be unconventional or uncomfortable. Taking action is stepping into discomfort. It also means you're seeking the suck, like my friend says. My perception for the Philly Half Marathon wasn't perfect, but because I took action, my reality changed. It changed immediately following the race weekend, and especially right after the weekend results were posted.

My question for you is: *What is your current reality?*

Your current reality is based on your current perception. *What's your perception of yourself?*

If you don't like your reality, it's time to change your perception by taking action. Think about your life and ask yourself: *How can I change my perception?*

You don't need to make a major change. In fact, I'd recommend starting small.

Are you willing to acknowledge the tension in your life and welcome the opportunity for growth in those weak points? That's what I determine to be perception. And that's why it's so important for athletes to understand the power of changing your perception. It's the only way you see growth.

What you think of yourself will always matter more than what others think of you! If you can control the climate on the inside of your life, then the outside climate doesn't need to be controlled. When it is summer outside, my wife and I are always asking each other to crank the AC. And it seems we are always saying to our daughter, "Brielle! Close the windows in your room right now, you're letting all the hot air in!" In life, you control your climate! It is an inside job. Set the internal temperature to whatever you need it to be set. Stop letting other people control your climate.

"I don't mean to say that I have already achieved these things or that I have already reached perfection. But I press on to possess that perfection for which Christ Jesus first possessed me."

— PHILIPPIANS 3:12 (NLT)

CHAPTER 11

Progress Over Perfection

RACE: 2014 STEELERS GATORADE 5K; RESULT: 22:18, MILE PACE 7:10/MI

What would you say if someone asked you to describe the best day of your life? Maybe you'd talk about graduation from high school or college. Maybe you'd talk about the day you proposed to your wife. Or maybe you'd say it was your wedding day or the day your child was born.

All of those are great answers, don't get me wrong. Those responses mark some of life's key milestones; each of those moments is filled with immense joy, gratefulness, and celebration. In fact, I can relate to a lot of those "best days," because I've also lived them. But those events have likely happened already—they are in the past. And the thing about the past is we can't go back and relive it, as nice as that sounds. We are only promised today.

What if we live for today instead of looking to the

past or trying to jump ahead to the future? What if you challenge yourself to have the best day ever—*today*?

What would that look like?

Living for today means leaning into the *progress over perfection* mindset.

The *progress over perfection* mindset keeps you in mental attack mode. *Progress over perfection* helps you focus on: competing with yourself, staying in your lane, and finding ways to grow. If you're living for today, there are plenty of opportunities for growth and much progress to be made. You acknowledge your best can be better, and you are willing to consistently take action to improve. *Progress over perfection* helps you see the little details you didn't notice before, which in turn helps you pivot into a better and brighter future.

Progress over perfection also means letting go of the idea of perfection: in school work, in athletic performances, and even in our relationships. We think perfection equals greatness, and *we want that*. But only Jesus Christ is perfect, and *we need to accept that*.

Is that something you are willing to accept?

The pressure to perform is having a perfectionistic mindset. If you have had a bad race and you're thinking about it from a perfectionistic mindset, you're setting yourself up to fail. If you haven't already, I encourage you to let go of this mindset. It's not real or attainable and will save you so much heartache.

Can you live for today and focus on making progress instead?

For every day I train, I know I've made progress: in my racing time, in my average mile pace, in my mental attitude . . . even in my nutrition, sleep habits, and daily routine. I've seen progress because I'm taking action rather than being inactive and afraid to start. Failure is worldly and, quite frankly, something that doesn't define me. My father, the Lord, defines who I am. He knows *progress over perfection* is more important because it provides me with opportunities for growth.

If you can accept that, there are only opportunities for winning and learning. Losses don't really exist, either. Rather, losses are seen as just smaller steps, strides, or pivots to the next win. When we put pressure on ourselves to perform, we live in the *results* and not the *effort*—we miss the chance for progress. I've learned to let go of the perfection mindset and have leaned into progress and growth. Be proud, not only because of your finishing time but also because of what you went through. As a result, expect to grow through what you go through.

One thing about me is I've always had a low resting heart rate. Some would go to great lengths in order to say my heart is the most athletic heart rate they've ever seen. It's simply been like that the majority of my life. After my brain injury in 2013, multiple scenarios were discussed as to what had potentially caused me to fall down the stairs on that fateful day. Was it an accident? A stroke? A seizure? Or maybe I had an issue with my heart and blood was not flowing quick enough through my body. This improper flow of blood could have caused dizziness and a fall. We have all these speculations of what could have caused the fall but still don't know, and we never will. At this point, I'm okay with not knowing. I am making it personal and no longer take it personally. I use to take my brain injury personally, letting the outside dictate my climate. It was guilt, shame, frustration . . . you name it. But when I made it personal, that's when I set the climate. If you have creativity in your life, then you can choose to be positive and always pivot to progress.

About a week before Labor Day in 2014, I had a loop recorder implanted into my chest to monitor my heart rate 24/7. My doctor at the time didn't want to insert a pacemaker instead because of my age and some other symptoms. I talked to the doctor and asked him if I could still run the Steelers Gatorade 5K over Labor Day weekend.

He said, "Yeah, sure, you can run. Just watch the stitches, ok? Don't go hard. Don't go all out. You don't want the stitching to open up."

This moment felt monumental for me because I had truly realized what *progress over perfection* actually meant. I knew I just had a loop record put in, but I also made a decision. One of the best pieces of advice I've ever received is: *Make a decision, and then make it the right decision.* I'm still working on following that advice today (that's part of the process). But I'm sharing this message with you too, because I think it could be helpful for you as you let faith grow, pursue your athletic goals, and follow your dreams.

Anyway, I made the decision to run the Steelers 5K, and I was looking forward to it. I decided to adjust my time goals due to the loop recorder procedure I received the week before. By doing that, taking a step back and being aware of my new expectations, I altered my finishing time and felt content in making a decision that was right for me. I decided that I was going to finish three minutes slower.

On September 1, 2014, I ran in the Steelers Gatorade 5K. I felt great. Not only did I beat the time I expected, but I beat the time I had pivoted from with a loop recorder in my chest. Talk about *progress over perfection* —whoa!

From that race on, I built the confidence to compete in more races, including half marathons. Ever since the 2014 Steelers Gatorade 5K, I've reflected on that race as a pivotal moment and reminder of how to place *progress over perfection*. Only you can decide if you want to run a 5K one week after having a loop recorder put in your chest, or run a half marathon eight weeks after a traumatic brain injury. It's your mindset, your growth, and your story. Make a decision, and then make it the right decision. Make a decision that in this next race, the next test, or the next event in your life, you're going to give it your best. If you do that consistently, and you are consistently consistent, you will absolutely see growth. All of those "nexts" become *progress over perfection*.

When I look back at the Steelers 5K, I always see my progress. If I don't make the race times that I want to get, I can also stop, look, and ask myself, "How was my effort based on the pivots that I made?" Adjust if you need to, but don't do it because of what others are telling you. Don't give into your own doubts, either. Don't get stuck three feet from the finish line. Keep going. Keep showing up. Keep making *progress over perfection*.

Progress over perfection is showing up over time, consistently, no matter what. That's what the Steelers Gatorade 5K did for me. It reminded me of the power of showing up. After the race, when the results came in, I was so happy with my time and how I performed. I started getting into the habit of looking back at my races and feeling proud of my accomplishments: showing up, making adjustments, and learning the lessons.

Progress over perfection is so important because it allows you to see growth. Sometimes it's hard to see that growth when you're in the middle of a tough time or a season of struggle. In my *progress over perfection* mindset, I realized what led to my disappointment the day after the Pittsburgh Marathon in 2023. I was disappointed because I didn't get what I wanted when I wanted it. I finished in three hours, eighteen minutes, and fourteen seconds. It was one of the best race days, weather-wise. You could call it "perfect race weather." When a runner has perfect weather, they usually expect a dream finish. Heading into the Pittsburgh

Marathon, I felt extremely confident a huge marathon personal record was coming.

In 2022, I ran three hours, seven minutes, and twenty seconds (which is my current marathon best). It poured a majority of that 2022 race. If I could run 3:07:20 in pouring rain, I figured I could definitely run another personal best in ideal running conditions. Here I was, going into this race thinking about perfecting running conditions and living in light of what I did back in 2022. That was the problem. You want to look at your past as progress that helps inform your expectations. But you don't want to bank on that past, or you will end up deflated.

Now, finishing at 3:18:14, I could have been devastated. That is so far off the ultimate marathon, but being so focused on that fact will crush you. If I sit and beat myself up at 3:18:14, my mind and body will shut down. It's all about progress! There's only winning and learning. So many people are giving it their all to get a sub 3:30 marathon. I'm doing them a disservice by sulking at a finish of 3:18:14. So, what do I do next? I keep taking action anyway. I'm consistent. I'm aware of my weaknesses. I work towards improving my weaknesses instead of downplaying them or avoiding them.

If you start a training run or a race with a progress mindset, you're committing to taking small steps each day in doing better and being better. Over time, this mindset will get you closer to your goals more quickly than aiming for perfection. Making progress is so much more rewarding than trying to be perfect. You have a better chance of being consistently consistent and reaching momentum in your life. You make no progress by simply having the perfect mindset and never getting started.

The Lord calls us to progress each day, too. He asks us to be obedient to Him. That allows faith to grow.

PART THREE

Emptying the Tank in Love

"The more you grow like this, the more productive and useful you will be in your knowledge of our Lord Jesus Christ."

— 2 PETER 1:8 (NLT)

CHAPTER 12

Growth is Optional

RACE: 2022 ERIE PRESQUE ISLE HALF
MARATHON; RESULT: 1:27:54, MILE PACE:
6:42/MI

I 've heard it said that change happens in our lives every 90 days. We want to make sure we're ready to embrace change, because it's going to come to us whether we welcome it or not.

Change is inevitable. Growth is optional.

"Growth is a choice." I will never forget when I heard Hall of Famer and wide receiver, Issac Bruce of the St Louis Rams, say this on a sports Spectrum podcast episode during Super Bowl week in 2018. I was on a treadmill at Planet Fitness. I can remember almost exactly which treadmill it was. That is how powerful someone else's wisdom can be. That knowledge has been a part of me for five-plus years now.

If given the opportunity to grow, I'd strongly recommend you take it. It might be the most powerful choice of your life. Choose growth now if you have not already.

Remember, the title of this book is *Let Faith Grow: Running Through Adversity*. Ensure your faith is growing, not the pressure to perform.

The pressure to perform sometimes grows because we don't let people in. Often, this pressure can grow when we don't surround ourselves with the right people. If you're the smartest person in the room, go find a new room.

One way growth is optional is that you have the choice to either surround yourself with influential people or people who drain you. Let people help you. Mentors, friends, teachers, parents, and coaches are all great examples of people who can guide you along your journey. You need to connect with people who are ahead of where you are. Surround yourself with people who want the best for you.

One of my mentors, Brandon Hayes, says, "I am just standing on the shoulders of giants."

He has said this many times, to the point it has resonated deeply with me. This is what mentors can do for your growth. They see the vision, because they have been through the thick of it. They will lift you up on their shoulders for you to see. It's like when my little one, Charlie, says, "I want to see" or "Daddy, I can't see." I then put her up on my shoulders, so she can see. Mentors help you grow by lifting you up when you can't see the way. I hope you have stood on the shoulders of giants or let someone stand on yours.

*Real quick tangent! Do not confuse this phrase with
"carrying people on your back."*

Jim Rohn said it best when he said, "You can help a thousand . . . but you can't carry three on your back."

Sometimes you have to say, "Get off my back."

Let's tie this in with paying attention to the tension in your life! Do you carry people on your back? It can be tough to differentiate when you are carrying someone versus when you allow someone to stand on your shoulders. The concept of your growth can be tied in with experiences I have talked about in great detail throughout this book. There is a difference between carrying someone on your back, and standing on the shoulders of giants. In fact, one will stunt your growth and create the wrong kind of tension in your life! This kind of tension will drain you. Pay attention to the details.

Growth also means you get so caught up in encouraging others that you encourage yourself. For others, your trial is blazing a trail. But, you've gone out of your way because someone blazed a trail for you in the midst of their trials. Drop your ego that thinks you can do life on your own. We are all in this together, and we need to make a commitment to each other.

At the beginning of my journey, I was going on my own. When I set goals to race, I thought it was just me on my own. I had an ego. I was a brain injury survivor. I wasn't vulnerable. I was trying to figure it out all alone. Don't be like me. Don't be so caught up in your training, goals, and the idea that you have to do everything on your own. Don't confuse having an ego with strength. Growth is optional, but it's not easy. When you grow, you will trust yourself and get excited. People will see that.

By choosing growth, you're being vulnerable. You're setting your ego aside and letting people into your life. But you are also being selective. This is a good thing—a *really* good thing. Sharing is caring. Let people into your life, and learn to be honest and vulnerable with trustworthy individuals.

Think about your relationships. Relationships are "ships." And ships are meant to go somewhere. If your relationships aren't moving, check it. If your relationships are moving to a place you don't like, check that, too. If you don't check them, your avoidance will only lead to tension. Don't do everything on your own. Having an ego and not being vulnerable will also lead to tension.

My story really started to change when I joined running groups. I started sharing my story with others, making me see people differently at races. Over the course of a few years people started inviting me to share my story on their podcasts. Having the platform to share my story was very emotional for me in a good way. I started to realize that my adversity is another person's blessing. Part of choosing growth meant committing to being uncomfortable and committing to adversity. I am asking you to commit to others. I noticed growth when I let mentors come into my life as well. As you've read, I've had a couple of coaches impact my mindset, too. When you're vulnerable and can let go of your ego, you allow for true change and growth to happen.

One year, I did a 5K not too far from my house on the trail. On the back half of the race, I'm finally neck and neck with this individual next to me. I know this individual won this 5K the year before, and we're both running hard. We're putting lots of effort into our race and pushing our bodies to their physical limits.

All of a sudden, for whatever reason, in my mind, I thought, "You know what? He deserves this. This guy deserves to win. I'm okay with second place."

So, I took my foot off the gas near the end of this 5K that I very likely could have won.

I said, "You know what? I'm going to coast in for a second-place finish. I can live with that."

I hadn't grown yet. My self-worth wasn't tied in with being a winner, which is mind-boggling because my goal is to be in the Olympics. Isn't that something? I didn't have enough self-worth to take first place in a local 5K, yet I want to go to the Olympics. That's growth, my friends.

Confidence is building the character you want to be. I wasn't where I wanted to be in that race.

With this mentality and by taking my foot off the gas, guess what happened? The two guys who were being who I wanted to be caught up. But I didn't see them. They caught up with me and passed me up. I finished, and I got a PR in the race. I felt great, but I gave up at the very end. I slowed down. This is a perfect example of living in the EFFORT and NOT THE RESULTS. Why?

My personal growth wasn't complete. My personal value was incomplete. At this point, early on in my racing career, I still had the brain injury mindset: "Dude, you had a brain injury. This is you. This is fantastic. You did so good. Second place, good for you. The person you're letting in front of you deserves it more than you."

When you compete, there's nothing wrong with giving it everything you've got. Competition is about making the competition better. I'll work on me for you if you work on you for you.

Jim Rohn could not have said it any better: "I don't like to win. For me, I wish for you to lose."

He says that because that's where growth is. There's winning and there's learning. Wisdom is your collective experience of winning and losing (I like to call it learning). Sometimes, you've got to win, so the other person loses and learns. The other person learns they have to give it everything that they have. Don't quit and settle for second place.

Now, when I go out and run, I'm not focused on the person that's second. I don't even focus on who is next to me or when we are going to finish.

In fact, at the 2022 Erie Presque Isle Half Marathon,

I got out quickly and efficiently at the start; I was feeling great. I didn't care about the weather. I didn't care about how hot it was.

I cared about only one thing: What I could control. Guess what I could control?

Me and my mindset. That's it. But it's just enough.

I'm at the starting line. I'm feeling great. The first group, Group A, shot out of the start like a cannon. I'm just behind Group A, and there's some really good, almost elite-level athletes going at a fast clip. I couldn't catch up to them. About six miles into the marathon, I'm in no man's land. I'm all by myself. But I feel good, and I'm not panicking. I'm not thinking about being all by myself. (In previous races, I have panicked, lost focus and made a wrong turn).

All of a sudden, out of nowhere, a gentleman comes up behind me. He would become a friend after this race. His name is Mike Urso. I want to thank him for one of the best race experiences of my life.

His sudden appearance made my instincts kick in, like, "Hey, you need to pick up the pace. You're behind elite Group A. You're probably not going to catch them, but you need to be consistent. You need to drop this guy who appeared out of nowhere. You're in a race."

Instead of giving in and giving the guy behind me the victory, I tried to lose him for a couple of miles. Finally, I realized I wasn't going to lose him. It wasn't in the cards. I ended up telling him, "Come on, let's go. Let's go together!" He comes up to me, and all of a sudden, without knowing each other, we became teammates for about five or six miles, maybe one-half of the 13.12-mile race . . . But we're neck and neck the whole time, keeping pace together. As we're going, he says to me, "I don't think I would be able to finish where I'm at if I wasn't running with you."

That's growth, my friend. I didn't let this other guy catch up to me because he deserved it more. Remember, I tried to drop him a couple of miles in. Then, I finally had him come join me, and we became one. Now, we're a team. We start picking off people I wouldn't have been able to pick off on my own.

After running about two miles together, he says, "Listen, I know you can run a lot faster. I can't go all out."

The last part of the thirteen-mile loop is a big hill. He knew I had a kick, and that I could finish stronger.

He said, "Whenever you're ready, take off."

I said, "Dude, I'm going to run with you as much as I can."

We kept running together. We helped each other keep pace. But the last mile or so, I ditched him. I kicked it up as opposed to the 5K a few years back where I let the kid next to me win the race. But I also knew there was so much growth in him and I running together to be able to pick off runners, change water stations, and be teammates.

Before I took off, he said, "Make sure you find me at the finish line."

I took off and finished the race, and, true to my word, I caught up with him after he finished the race.

There was so much growth in my self-esteem from deciding to run with him. I didn't let him win, but we joined forces and became friends. I wouldn't have done that if I didn't have a growth-oriented mindset. I would have let him pass me if I hadn't taken the opportunity to grow and learn from my choices at the 5K. The pattern would have continued and repeated. But rather than doing that, I chose growth.

Side note: This is the Erie Presque Isle Half Marathon. And if you remember the name of the race, I did a full marathon in the past where I tripped on my dang shoelace at Mile 18. Remember that? Ha! I sure remember it. Now here I am running one of the best races on the same course. I'm just here on a different day.

Change is going to happen. To think differently is naive, but you'll grow through what you go through, both the good and the bad. If you want to be consistently consistent, or make progress over perfection in this life, you have to grasp the idea that growth is optional. You also have to find ways to grow each day in some way. When you choose growth, you're choosing to make it personal, not take it personally. That's growth.

We met up afterwards, and I got to meet his wife. I found out that they have a beautiful little girl who's about the same age as my youngest daughter, Charlie. I learned about where he works and what he does for a living. I even found out that they lived in the neighbor-hood that I had grown up in. We have become good friends ever since that race.

In fact, one of my best racing photos I've ever obtained was taken by Mike's mother-in-law. She took a photo of us running side by side. We were two total strangers who'd never met before. But if you look at the photo, it feels like the two people in it have been teammates for years. It is as if we grew up to be training buddies.

The last piece of wisdom I'll leave you with is that when you choose growth and really allow that to become your mindset, it's an inside job. A lot of times, you'll have growth before you see progress. Progress over perfection. You can feel progress before anyone else ever sees it. When you feel progress, it's actually growth. Growth becomes confidence and belief in yourself . . . You grow on the inside, even if you can't see it.

The bigger a tree is, the harder it is to get knocked down because the roots are so deep and ingrained into the ground. You want to have good habits that run deep, sort of like tree roots. Seeing our habits from the outside is tough, but we can feel them within. Growth is the progress we feel. That's going to give you momentum when you make a decision. When you choose to grow, the first thing you should do is set your goals, set your day, your month, and your life. Remember, growth is optional. It's up to you.

You have the choice to grow, choice to love, choice

to be vulnerable, choice to open up. Isn't that powerful? Choose to let people in. Choose to share your story. Your mess is a message. Your adversity is meant to bless others. Your trial is a trail for someone else. I'm asking you to choose growth, today and always.

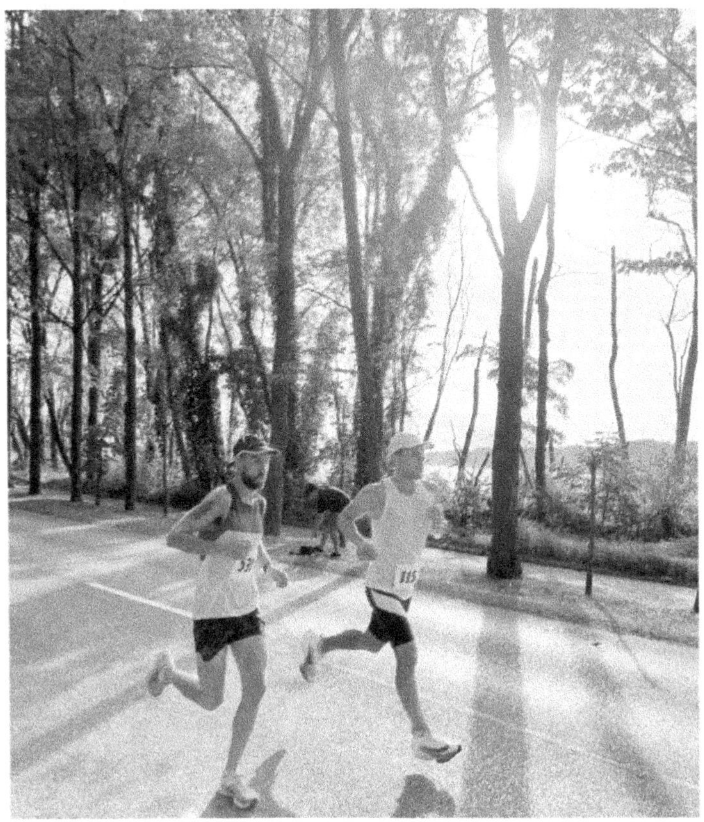

Mike Urso and I running together at the 2022 Erie Presque Isle Half Marathon.

"Through Jesus, therefore, let us continually offer to God a sacrifice of praise—the fruit of lips that openly profess his name. And do not forget to do good and to share with others, for with such sacrifices God is pleased."

— HEBREWS 13:15-16

Epilogue

It has been twelve years since I really began wanting to compete as an Olympic athlete. The seed was planted sometime in July of 2012 in my driveway. My journey and progress have continued to shine and grow in that timeframe, but I feel like there's still so much more I need to do to get there. God is a last-minute miracle worker. Just stay obedient and true.

My goal is to qualify for the 2024 Olympics at the Chicago International Marathon. That's the plan as of now (God will have the final say in that plan), but I'll be ready to pivot when the time comes. Ironically, that's also the last day to qualify for the Olympic Trials. I will live with a chance of failure and then with regret! That's the mindset. That date might seem far away, but it's really much closer than it seems. The challenge is I need to cut one hour off of my current time, which is my 3:18 showing at the Pittsburgh Marathon. I know I have to put in the work and keep progressing each day. I have to *think, act, adjust,* and *try again.* I must apply the principles in this book to keep pivoting, moving and growing. I'm also trusting the Lord to guide my steps as I train and *put my plans in sand.* If you're curious on how things turn out, you can follow me on my Instagram at @let_faith_grow. I'd love to hear from you!

Before you close this book, I want to leave you with a couple more thoughts. First, life is 90% mental and 10% physical. Your attitude and mental outlook will guide you throughout your life. This whole book is all about what you can do, the conversations you have with yourself, and the mental shifts that only you have the choice to make. You'll see true progress when the internal game (your mindset) changes. I guarantee it.

The last thing I'd like to impart to you is feel free to use the principles in this book in the best way that works for you, wherever you're at in your journey. Test them out, and make them your own. But don't feel like you have to follow them in a certain order. They all work together, but at the end of the day, my guidance here is more about wanting you to believe in yourself and giving you practical ways you can help your faith grow. When you *let faith grow,* you can *let fear go.*

I BELIEVE IN YOU. LET FAITH GROW (LFG).

— Ben Hinton

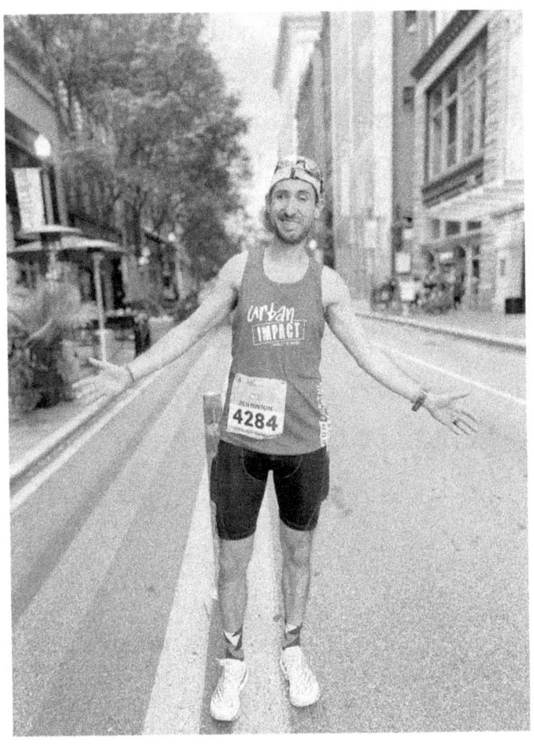

Ben Hinton resides right outside of Pittsburgh, Pennsylvania, with his wife, two kids, and their family dog (Atlantis) of nine years. (And, they are adopting a new puppy in July of 2023!) Ben is passionate about teaching people about faith, the pressure to perform, and a growth mindset which he covers in his book through themes such as *progress over perfection* and pivoting by *putting your plans in the sand*. After having sustained a brain injury as a young adult, he has turned his life experiences into messages of hope. He aims to reveal hope in the midst of trial by running through adversity. He spent several years as a youth basketball coach. He also has previous experience as a Paraprofessional working with the autistic and life skills support. He has been chasing very audacious running goals in the marathon distance since 2013 and hopes to soon qualify for the Olympics. Thanks be to God, Ben's philosophy is, "Be encouraged every day and let faith grow."

To get in touch with Ben, you can follow his social media handle @let_faith_grow or email him at <u>beencouragedeveryday@gmail.com</u>.

Acknowledgments

I keep telling people the hardest part of this book so far has been the acknowledgment section. I have made several calls and have sent messages to various people reminding them how much I appreciate them being a part of my journey. I was even talking to my friend from Japan, and we talked about the pros and cons of keeping the acknowledging section short. I thought I made up my mind to do just that, but yet here I am not keeping it short one bit.

One of the best pieces of advice I have ever got was "Make a decision and make it the right decision."

So, I am going to do just that with this acknowledgment. I apologize in advance to anyone who I didn't thank, but they felt they deserved a thanks. I recommend you sit down and try writing or typing an acknowledgment section. You don't need the intention of writing a book or showing it to anyone. I simply believe when you sit down and write out an "acknowledgment" it can be very therapeutic. It makes you realize people have had an impact on your life whether the impact lasted 30 seconds, 30 days, or 30 years. I could have chosen to make the section short and sweet and thank just the incredible people who had a hand in this book. Everyone has had a hand in this book when it comes down to it, because somehow and someway, everyone has impacted me. This book is me sharing my journey.

I am not trying to speak for all brain injury survivors. I will speak for myself as I struggled with feeling disconnected for a long time after my brain injury. When you have a significant brain injury as an adult, you struggle with the past, present, and future. You carry so much guilt and confusion. I will tell you the good news: Time doesn't necessarily "heal" all wounds, but you can get stronger and grow through what you go through or have been through. That is what makes these acknowledgments so personal for me (*make it personal, don't take it personally*). I am making it personal so I can attempt to express how thankful I am for everyone. I want to emphasize here just how connected we all are. I have met so many people through so many other people, organically or inorganically. Remember that life is in the details and the details are in God.

I want to thank my Lord and Savior, Jesus Christ. He sacrificed His life for mine. I want to also thank my mom and dad. While I do not have a relationship with my dad, I still am thankful for him. I want to thank my mom for doing the best she could with the cards she was dealt. She successfully raised me as a single mom. She sacrificed so much for me.

I have to thank my wife because I still try to process

everything she has been through during the almost ten years of our marriage and beyond that. To go from being engaged and then roughly six months later you find your fiancé on the stairs when you get home from work, to soon find out he had been fighting consciousness for four hours. I still can't imagine. Because this journey has been nothing short of difficult for me, it has taken so much from her and of her at times. She is my driving force. I am so incredibly thankful for her. It has been a lot. I am also thankful for those who have stepped in and supported her at times she felt I couldn't or didn't support her. She has helped raise two of the best little girls. I have at times been complimented as a father, but Crystal and my in-laws are the biggest reason for the girls' success.

I want to thank so many other families. They have been vital in planting the seed into who I needed to be in my formative years and have helped develop me into who I am today. Those families include the Tichota family and the Poremba family. Looking back, I spent time around the Tichota family with many fond memories until just before I was nine years old. I was embraced by their love and hospitality. I grew up with their sons Clay and Ross, and I couldn't imagine growing up around better kids in those years and being lucky to see their families grow now as I head into my soon-to-be 40's. The Poremba family took me in during my elementary years and beyond. I always lived with my mom on my grandparents' family property. My second family was literally the Porembas.

Matt and Mike have grown up to be incredibly successful, and are now husbands and fathers. They had
world-class examples in their parents, John and
Beverly.

I want to thank the Nedele family, Brad in particular! Like the Poremba brothers, Matt and Mike, Brad is
a "friend" who is also family. Both Brad and the
Poremba brothers fit into the "when your friends
become family" group. I have been so thankful to have
stayed connected with Brad and the Porembas long
enough. It is a blessing that we've been able to grow
up together through so many milestones: school, our
20s, our weddings, and now we're raising kids. I am
also lucky to say I get along with all three of their
wives and can call them just as good of friends. I
cannot leave out Mark, either. He still looks and acts
like he did the day we first met. I can't even tell you
how old he is. I hope you continue to never age,
buddy.

I have to give a special shoutout to my friend,
Danny Fernandez. I met Danny in college as I was
sitting in a Starbucks directly off campus nearby where
I used to live. After that brief chat about Apple laptops,
I would find out that we would end up creating a
friendship that still lasts to this day. He eventually had
to move to Japan to go to Carnegie Mellon University
because his visa could not be extended for him to finish
his dissertation. We still chat often, because his conversations always make me feel I have gained worldly
knowledge. He always challenges my perspective, or

gives me a tip that helps me grow as a person. He does all of this so casually.

This is where the acknowledgments got really hard for me: when I thought about thanking my doctors. I have seen so many doctors over the years that I unfortunately have forgotten some of their names.

These are doctors that saved my life. I have had some incredible doctors who have literally poured their life, time, and purpose into my life and survival.

I have to give a special shoutout to my aforementioned friend, Dr. Poremba.

Thank you to Dr. Andrew Eller out of the Pittsburgh Eye and Ear Institute. He can be credited with my ability to even see at all.

I have to thank Dr. Jeffrey Liu. He inserted a loop recorder in my chest in 2014. A loop recorder keeps track of your heart rate 24/7. We decided to put in a loop recorder because he wanted to be able to monitor my heart, but he didn't want me to have a pacemaker. He truly got who I was and understood my passion and need for running. He listened to me, trusted me, and encouraged me to live the lifestyle I was living.

Thank you to Dr. Collins, who oversaw a lot after my brain injury and followed me from the concussion protocol, medication, and rehab for quite some time. I will never remember the first time I walked into his office.

He asked me, "What brings you here?"

I told him a little bit and then he couldn't believe I was able to physically walk, let alone walk into his office. He was just another doctor who validated me in how I was trying to live my life moving forward.

I have to give special thanks to all the therapists who have crossed paths with me over the years. I have worked with so many over the years because of my balance system (vestibular) being shattered from my accident in 2013.

I would like to give a very brief, but important thanks to someone in particular, Paul Dooley. He was working as an aid with brain injury survivors. He used to just talk to me. There was a time during my recovery when I felt like I was always being talked at and not talked with. When it comes to mental health, I feel that is a narrative many struggle with. The frustration of trying to explain how you feel, but people not always understanding you. People do listen and can understand. A few simple conversations with him helped shape my life moving forward after the toughest day of my life. That is why they are conversations I will never forget during breaks between therapy sessions or over lunch breaks.

I have had some amazing personal trainers over the years as well. I want to give a shoutout to Julius Scott. He is someone I worked with before my accident. I worked with him a lot when I first got out of college and still thought basketball was the direction I was heading. We worked out hard. I was only able to go hard because we trusted each other and pushed each other. That energy grew into a great friendship.

There are two other trainers and coaches that I

really need to give acknowledgment to. I started working with Dee in the summer of 2012. I was able to be upfront with her and tell her my huge audacious goals. She was on board for it. We did so much work together. When I survived my brain injury in 2013, they always attributed my age and my fitness as to why I survived. I got in better shape the older I have become because I have learned more about the process. A major part of the process is that you want to push yourself and work when no one is watching. The other half of that is getting around people who will help push you beyond your limits and keep you accountable.

There is a saying that relates to this which is: "If you want to go fast, go alone, if you want to go far, go together."

Dee is who I went back to after my brain injury. I wanted to push myself.

Have you ever been told to "work harder on yourself than you do on your job"?

I needed to return to work because Dee was putting me in the best place to succeed and grow. I did a lot of physical therapy when I did my brain rehabilitation. I often got very frustrated because PT rehab gave me tasks that were mundane and not very challenging like the things I was already doing with Dee.

Kamden Hofflman and her husband are two other people that need to be acknowledged. Kamden was such a great triathlon coach in the Pittsburgh area. In my first ever 5K, she also ran in the event. It was the first event I had a smartwatch on and really had someone measure my progress. I will never forget her screaming my name on the course whistle. She was also a participant on the course. I finished that first 5K in around 27 minutes. My current 5K racing PR is 18:35. You can tell how much of an impact her encouragement was for that first 5k and beyond. She didn't stop there. She cheered me on during my first indoor triathlon event. She didn't just coach me. She cheered me on. I don't know for certain when the two-mile sprint was at the end of the event, but it was around the sixth mile on that loop track, because I could hear her.

In 2016, I started working as a paraprofessional in the Bethel Park School District.

I have so many to give thanks to from the faculty: Mr. Muench and Dr. Spararlis, who became my mentors, gave me confidence, gave me a chance, and really took care of my own safety several times, to the staff I was fortunate to work with; Bill Javor, Mr. Staranko, Jen O'neal, Mrs. Ragatti, Mrs. W, and Surrena Lynn. I learned so much from getting to watch Surrena Lynn as a speech therapist. I was able to learn from her interactions with kids. I worked with Mrs. W (Susan) for one year; when she first came to our building and became a para in town, I felt she looked familiar to me. It turned out that we attended the same church. As the year went out, we became good friends and she really catapulted me into writing a book. It is something I wanted to do for a while, but she really convinced me.

I can't forget Mrs. Barret and Diane Jacobson.

Sandy Blacknore was also a huge influential person.

She was one of the most helpful people I have ever worked with. She was my training. As a paraprofessional, you can get thrown into the fire. She was someone that just automatically took me under her wing.

I know I missed mentioning some of the faculty I was so honored to learn from as a paraprofessional.

I also had the privilege to coach some young talented junior high athletes on the 7th and 8th-grade basketball team for a few years at Bethel. I'm thankful for that experience. That was my last time coaching a team. I walked away from coaching because I knew I could really only give my personal attention to running. I wanted to commit to coaching basketball, but it didn't pan out. Sometimes part of growth is knowing who and what you can commit to and why. That time coaching them was extremely impactful to me.

I want to thank the love and support I witnessed parents and families give their children, especially from the Stromberg and Holzer families.

I worked one year with Carrie Holzer's son. And it was a year I will never forget.

If you are a parent, paraprofessional, or just need a good book please, I beg of you . . . pick up a copy of her book *Building Puzzles Underwater: An Autism Story*. This was one of the best books I have ever read.

Working as a paraprofessional in life skills and autistic support, parents taught me that "no one will ever be your biggest advocate besides you."

Parents whose children are diagnosed with Autism advocate for their kids more than anyone I have ever seen do so. Many times I saw true growth in the parents who taught their children how to advocate for themselves. I took on a personal challenge to get students to become independent. This experience has really helped me as a parent myself.

The Fabus family needs to be mentioned as well. They created the Fabus Foundation after the passing of their son, Joey Fabus. He passed because of an incurable childhood brain cancer. They hold an annual 5K in Joey's honor and the way the Bethel Park Community shows up each year is astounding. It always touches me. Both Joey and his parents are superheroes in my eyes.

As you know, growing up, many years were spent at the local YMCA that was essentially one of my second homes. There were so many mentors I grew up with that I will tell you shaped my life. In particular, Jeff Spinelli, Billy Selko, the Clark brothers, Kyle Witucki, Joe Lunchino, and many others helped a young kid grow up through some pretty difficult times. Joe actually became an assistant coach with me when I had my first coaching gig for a 3rd-4th grade team and 5th-6th grade team in a diocese school just outside of Pittsburgh. Having him as an assistant coach with me was one of my best coaching memories.

I have to also thank the Dezort Family in those early coaching years.

I will never forget my time coaching the girls team at St. Elizabeth, thanks to the athletic director at the time, Mr. Richardson, and my parent assistant, Mr. Myers. I enjoyed working with that program so much. They were such hard workers, and they were some of the best parents a coach could work with. Let's be honest, that isn't always the coach's sentiments when it comes to parents, ha.

I have to give a thank you to Coach Colombo who was my basketball coaching mentor. I still call him coach and I always will. A special shoutout to Justin Policie who introduced me to coach Colombo. Justin's son is now a phenomenal young player! Justin and I had a phone call not too long ago. Justin thought Coach Colombo and I would hit it off, and we sure did.

I was part of the Players Edge camp and program developed for younger basketball athletes around the greater Pittsburgh area. The Players Edge Association also helped me land more coaching in the AAU circuit. The Players Edge is also where I met Josh Rulnik. We strengthened our friendship over the last several years as we both have transitioned from the basketball world into the running world.

I have to give a special shoutout to the entire running community that I have become friends with over the years. A special shoutout to all my friends over at the Facebook group, the Boston Buddies. A special shoutout to what Scott Rieke has done with his Ordinary Marathoners group organically over the years (the group developed into a nonprofit foundation and his Ordinary Marathoners podcast). The online running group, Iron Sharpens Iron, has been great. Jesse Wililams has created some of the best Facebook running groups that are centered around faith.

Dennis Morris is a friend I met through the running community online. One day she sent me a copy of Ryian Hall's book, *Run the Mile You're In*. She said this book reminded her of me. She got a signed copy when she briefly met Ryan at a book signing. Have I said, "Life is in the details and the details are in God"? After reading that book I wanted to be trained by Ryan Hall. This was even more so after I saw his running documentary "The 41st Day". I highly recommend that running documentary!

Lo and behold I would end up training with Ryan Hall. (Check the front cover of this book.) So, Thank you to my running coaches, including Jimmy Stevens, and the founders of the Run Free Online coaching platform: Ryan Hall, Jay Stepehon, Mitch Robertson, and the entire Run Free family of coaches and athletes. Along with running and supplementing, I have been enjoying 6AM Run Nutrition. I have been honored to get to know the CEO, Hami Mahani. In my experience the customer service, culture, and product from 6AM Run has been amazing.

I also want to give a special thanks to a few authors who I have been privileged to say are my friends and mentors as well. Jeremey Taylor, Greg Walker, Matt Scoletti, and Melvin Banks are just a few. What has been amazing is the friendships forged just out of knowing those individuals. My plan was to run in the 2023 Houston Marathon, which was January 15, 2023. I was going to use it to see where I was at with my fitness and then pivot the rest of my races in 2023 as an attempt to get the qualifying standard time for the 2024 Olympic Trials. I didn't get to that starting line in Houston. God had another plan for me. I ended up meeting Adam F. Jones, a leader and author in the Pittsburgh area. Going to his seminar in Pittsburgh the weekend of the Houston Marathon changed the trajectory and growth for me in many needed ways.

I know this is the longest acknowledgement and I truly thank you for reading this. I can't tell you how much I appreciate you taking time out of your life to spend it with me.

I have to give an acknowledgment to the entire Streamline Books team. Thank you to Nathan Sahly, Will Severns, and Alex Demczak. I felt we became friends on day one. We had group text chats going so fast. Or maybe it's because I created group chats so fast and they just came along, ha. I have to tell you I wouldn't have ever signed to be an author with Streamline if it wasn't for Alex Demczak. I heard Alex share his story on a Sports Spectrum Podcast. In that episode, he shared his story of sports and faith. He shared how he became a QB on the Missouri Tigers D1 Football team. He was led to follow a world-renowned author and speaker, Jon Gordon. I had been reading Jon Gordon's books for years. Side note: Coach Scott Colombo gave me my first Jon Gordon book years ago. Alex wrote a book with Jon called *The Sale*. It is a fable about a salesman and his journey with integrity. It is a phenomenal book.

After hearing Alex's story on the podcast I heard he started the company, Streamline Books. I reached out to Alex via Instagram. The rest is history (I am saying this to keep a long acknowledgment no longer).

I remember chatting with Nathan on the phone. His incredible personality and genuine nature got me on board with the team. The team at Streamline knows how much I have loved doing this and I have grown in this journey with them. I threw LFG around so much in emails, texts, and video calls that the title had to be *Let Faith Grow*.

Then I met and worked with Allison Lewis who became my ghostwriter for this book. She has made this the best experience and process of my life. Her writing, listening skills, and faith are what made this book. She has literally taken the words out of my mouth and placed them directly into this book.

I am forever thankful for the professionalism of Trevor Waite who was flawless as the book team manager.

I am thankful for Will, the other co-founder of Streamline Books, who has always spoken life into any conversation he has had. I have gotten to know both Alex and Will personally. I am so thankful to be around other men with young kids who I know will help me to continue to grow.

We see athletes of all ages yelling LFG. We know what they are mouthing when they scream out LFG. The viewers can read their lips. I have since and I want to start a new trend for athletes. I would like to change the meaning behind LFG. I cannot wait to hear athletes yelling "LET FAITH GROW" at the top of their lungs for everyone. Because after all, this journey is always bigger than one of us.

By the way, Jason Romano used to be a former ESPN player years ago. Tony Dungy spoke highly of Jason Romano in a book called *Uncommon*. I read that book. I followed Jason on Twitter. It turns out he took a job as an executive at Sports Spectrum at the intersection of faith and sports. I have since been blessed to get to know Jason some. With that, LFG Thank you and God bless you.